# Surgical Palliative Care and Pain Management

*Guest Editors*

GEOFFREY P. DUNN, MD
SUGANTHA GANAPATHY, MBBS
VINCENT CHAN, MD

# ANESTHESIOLOGY CLINICS

www.anesthesiology.theclinics.com

*Consulting Editor*
LEE A. FLEISHER, MD, FACC

March 2012 • Volume 30 • Number 1

SAUNDERS an imprint of ELSEVIER, Inc.

**W.B. SAUNDERS COMPANY**
*A Division of Elsevier Inc.*

1600 John F. Kennedy Boulevard, Suite 1800 ● Philadelphia, PA 19103-2899

http://www.theclinics.com

**ANESTHESIOLOGY CLINICS Volume 30, Number 1**
**March 2012 ISSN 1932-2275, ISBN-13: 978-1-4557-4208-0**

Editor: Rachel Glover

*Anesthesiology Clinics* (ISSN 1932-2275) is published quarterly by Elsevier Inc., 360 Park Avenue South, New York, NY 10010-1710. Months of issue are March, June, September, and December. Periodicals postage paid at New York, NY and at additional mailing offices. Subscription prices are $154.00 per year (US student/resident), $313.00 per year (US individuals), $383.00 per year (Canadian individuals), $496.00 per year (US institutions), $615.00 per year (Canadian institutions), $216.00 per year (Canadian and foreign student/resident), $434.00 per year (foreign individuals), and $615.00 per year (foreign institutions). To receive student and resident rate, orders must be accompanied by name of affiliated institution, date of term, and the *signature* of program/residency coordinator on institutions letterhead. Orders will be billed at individual rate until proof of status is received. Foreign air speed delivery is included in all *Clinics'* subscription prices. All prices are subject to change without notice. POSTMASTER: Send address changes to *Anesthesiology Clinics,* Elsevier Health Sciences Division, Subscription Customer Service, 3251 Riverport Lane, Maryland Heights, MO 63043. Customer Service (orders, claims, online, change of address): Elsevier Health Sciences Division, Subscription Customer Service, 3251 Riverport Lane, Maryland Heights, MO 63043. Tel:1-800-654-2452 (U.S. and Canada); 314-447-8871 (outside U.S. and Canada). Fax: 314-447-8029. E-mail: journalscustomerservice-usa@elsevier.com (for print support); journalsonlinesupport-usa@elsevier.com (for online support).

*Reprints.* For copies of 100 or more of articles in this publication, please contact the Commercial Reprints Department, Elsevier Inc., 360 Park Avenue South, New York, NY 10010-1710. Tel.: 212-633-3812; Fax: 212-462-1935; E-mail: reprints@elsevier.com.

*Anesthesiology Clinics,* is also published in Spanish by McGraw-Hill Inter-americana Editores S. A., P.O. Box 5-237, 06500 Mexico D. F., Mexico.

*Anesthesiology Clinics*, is covered in *MEDLINE/PubMed (Index Medicus), Current Contents/Clinical Medicine, Excerpta Medica, ISI/BIOMED,* and *Chemical Abstracts.*

Printed and bound by CPI Group (UK) Ltd, Croydon, CR0 4YY

Transferred to Digital Print 2012

# Contributors

## CONSULTING EDITOR

**LEE A. FLEISHER, MD, FACC**
Robert D. Dripps Professor and Chair of Anesthesiology and Critical Care, University of Pennsylvania School of Medicine, Philadelphia, Pennsylvania

## GUEST EDITORS

**GEOFFREY P. DUNN, MD, FACS**
Department of Surgery and Palliative Care Consultation Service, UPMC Hamot Medical Center, Erie, Pennsylvania

**SUGANTHA GANAPATHY, MBBS, DA, FRCA, FFARCS (I), FRCPC**
Professor of Anesthesiology and Perioperative Medicine, Director of Regional and Pain Research, Department of Anesthesiology and Perioperative Medicine, London Health Sciences Centre, University Hospital, University of Western Ontario, London, Ontario, Canada; Consulting Professor, Duke University Medical Centre, Durham, North Carolina

**VINCENT CHAN, MD, FRCPC**
Professor, Department of Anesthesiology, University of Toronto, Toronto Western Hospital, Toronto, Ontario, Canada

## AUTHORS

**PATRICK K. BIRMINGHAM, MD, FAAP**
Department of Pediatric Anesthesiology, Children's Memorial Hospital, Northwestern University's Feinberg School of Medicine, Chicago, Illinois

**ASOKUMAR BUVANENDRAN, MD**
Professor and Director of Orthopedic Anesthesia, Department of Anesthesiology, Rush University Medical Center, Chicago, Illinois

**JACQUES E. CHELLY, MD, PhD, MBA**
Professor of Anesthesiology (with Tenure) and Orthopedic Surgery; Vice Chair of Clinical Research; Director, Division of Acute Interventional Perioperative Pain and Regional Anesthesia; Director, Regional Anesthesia Fellowship, Department of Anesthesiology, University of Pittsburgh Medical Center, Pittsburgh, Pennsylvania

**GEOFFREY P. DUNN, MD, FACS**
Department of Surgery and Palliative Care Consultation Service, UPMC Hamot Medical Center, Erie, Pennsylvania

**JONATHAN R. GAVRIN, MD**
Physician Co-Chair, HUP Ethics Committee, Department of Anesthesiology and Critical Care, Hospital of the University of Pennsylvania, Philadelphia, Pennsylvania

**JOAN L. HUFFMAN, MD, FACS, CWS, FACCWS**
Medical Director, Wound Healing Program; Assistant Professor, Division of Acute Care
Surgery, Department of Surgery, University of Florida at Shands Jacksonville,
Jacksonville, Florida

**RYAN J. KOZLOWSKI, BS**
Medical Student, Department of Pediatric Anesthesiology, Children's Memorial Hospital,
Northwestern University's Feinberg School of Medicine, Chicago, Illinois

**THOMAS J. MINER, MD**
Assistant Professor of Surgery, Associate Program Director, General Surgery; Director
of Surgical Oncology, Department of Surgery, The Alpert Medical School of Brown
University, Rhode Island Hospital, Providence, Rhode Island

**ANNE CHARLOTTE MOSENTHAL, MD, FACS**
Professor of Surgery, New Jersey Medical School, University of Medicine and Dentistry
of New Jersey, Newark, New Jersey

**THOMAS H. SCOTT, MD**
Fellow in Pain Management, Department of Anesthesiology and Critical Care, Perelman
School of Medicine, University of Pennsylvania, Philadelphia, Pennsylvania

**SANTHANAM SURESH, MD, FAAP**
Professor of Anesthesiology and Pediatrics, Department of Pediatric Anesthesiology,
Children's Memorial Hospital, Northwestern University's Feinberg School of Medicine,
Chicago, Illinois

**CHRISTINE C. TOEVS, MD, FACS, FCCM**
Trauma Surgery, Surgical Critical Care, and Palliative Medicine, Allegheny General
Hospital, Pittsburgh, Pennsylvania

**LESLIE STEELE TYRIE, MD**
Assistant Professor of Surgery, New Jersey Medical School, University of Medicine and
Dentistry of New Jersey, Newark, New Jersey

**ADAM YOUNG, MD**
Resident, Department of Anesthesiology, Rush University Medical Center, Chicago,
Illinois

# Contents

> Palliative care in the United States has made tremendous strides in the last decade. One of the most perplexing issues arises when a palliative care patient presents to the operating room with an already existing do-not-resuscitate (DNR) order. This article describes the most common conflicting issues that may arise and provides guidance to surgeons, anesthesiologists, patients, and their primary physicians to reach satisfactory resolution and optimal care. Anesthesia departments should appoint a liaison to surgical and perioperative nursing departments to provide education and create an atmosphere conducive to discussions with palliative care patients about goals of care, including DNR status.

> Palliation has been an essential, if not the primary, activity of surgery during much of its history. However, it has been only during the past decade that the modern principles and practices of palliative care developed in the nonsurgical specialties in the United States and abroad have been introduced to surgical institutions, widely varied practice settings, education, and research.

> The purpose of palliative medicine is to prevent and relieve suffering and to help patients and their families set informed goals of care and treatment. Palliative medicine can be provided along with life-prolonging treatment or as the main focus of treatment. Increasingly, palliative medicine has a role in the surgical intensive care unit (SICU) and trauma. Data show involving palliative medicine in the SICU results in decreased length of stay, improved communication with families and patients, and earlier setting of goals of care, without increasing mortality. The use of triggers for palliative medicine consultation improves patient-centered care in the SICU.

**Recent Advances in Multimodal Analgesia**                                    91

Adam Young and Asokumar Buvanendran

> Greater understanding of the pathophysiology and mechanism of acute
> pain has led to advances in pharmacologic therapy. Understanding the
> principles of multimodal therapy along with surgical-specific protocols
> leads to improved outcome in patients. However, further large-scale ran-
> domized trials need to be performed to further establish and demonstrate
> the long-term benefit of multimodal therapy for patients undergoing
> surgery.

**Pediatric Pain Management**                                                 101

Santhanam Suresh, Patrick K. Birmingham, and Ryan J. Kozlowski

> Regional anesthesia has become an integral part of adult anesthesia.
> Although not routinely used in children because of the need for general an-
> esthesia that is necessary to keep the patients from moving and cooperat-
> ing with the operator, regional anesthesia has been gaining immense
> popularity in the last decade. Although there is not much objective
> evidence, large prospective databases and expert opinion have favored
> administering regional anesthesia in the asleep child safely because major
> neural damage has not been reported in children. This review discusses
> a comprehensive approach to acute pain management in infants, children,
> and adolescents using regional anesthesia.

**Index**                                                                      119

**VISIT US ONLINE!**
Access your subscription at:
**www.theclinics.com**

# Foreword

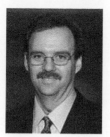

Lee A. Fleisher, MD
*Consulting Editor*

As anesthesiologists, we continue to strive to define old and new areas of cover in which we can demonstrate our value. One potential area of expansion for the anesthesiologist in the era of the Affordable Care Act is the concept of the surgical home. Palliative care is becoming a more important component of care for the surgical patient. As hospitals focus on preventable deaths, the delivery of palliative care has taken on increased importance. In this issue of *Anesthesiology Clinics*, we have been able to publish some outstanding articles from a recent issue of *Surgical Clinics*, as well as a new article related to anesthesia services related to palliative care, from an excellent group of leaders in the field.

As guest editor for this issue, we are fortunate to have Geoffrey P. Dunn, MD. Dr Dunn received his professional training at Jefferson Medical College and the New England Deaconess Hospital. He served as medical director of the Palliative Care Consultation Service and Great Lakes Hospice at Hamot. Since 1997, his work has focused on the education of surgeons nationally about the principles and practice of palliative care in the setting of serious and life-limiting illness. He is cochairman of the Surgical Palliative Care task force of the American College of Surgeons and was the editor of a monthly palliative care series that appeared in the *Journal of the American College of Surgeons*. He has assembled a stellar group of authors who provide important information for the anesthesiologist to understand an increasingly important component of our care, which can impact patient outcomes.

Lee A. Fleisher, MD
University of Pennsylvania School of Medicine
3400 Spruce Street, Dulles 680
Philadelphia, PA 19104, USA

E-mail address:
lee.fleisher@uphs.upenn.edu

Anesthesiology Clin 30 (2012) ix
doi:10.1016/j.anclin.2012.02.002
1932-2275/12/$ – see front matter

# SECTION 1:
# Surgical Palliative Care

Edited by Geoffrey P. Dunn, MD

# Preface

# Update on Surgical Palliative Care

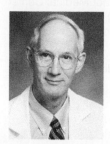

Geoffrey P. Dunn, MD
*Guest Editor*

Over the last decade, palliative care principles and practices have been increasingly recognized and integrated into the practice and institutions of surgery and anesthesia. During this time, the more general field of palliative care has established itself as a medical subspecialty and has created a high educational standard for itself through the establishment of over sixty fellowship programs and numerous other educational initiatives. Basic research is rapidly proliferating, although still lags in funding appropriate for the potential benefits. Hospital palliative care programs are rapidly proliferating while the National Quality Forum has identified quality indicators and best practices. Despite the recent political setback of the "death panel" characterization of federal funding for the most innocent of all medical interventions, the patient/doctor discussion about end-of-life treatment preferences, favorable public perception of palliative care is increasing, in part, due to the popular writings of surgeons Pauline Chen and Atul Gawande. Palliative care has become a timely lens through which the socioeconomic and spiritual bankruptcy of the current health care system and our prevailing expectations of the health care system are starkly visible especially when it is focused on the hospital care of patients with advanced and critical illness.

This volume demonstrates the diversity of application of the fundamental principles of palliative care to varied surgical specialties and settings. The articles have been selected to provide more depth to the philosophical and spiritual basis for this

A version of this article was published in the 91:2 issue of *Surgical Clinics of North America*.

Anesthesiology Clin 30 (2012) xiii–xiv
doi:10.1016/j.anclin.2011.11.006
1932-2275/12/$ – see front matter
**anesthesiology.theclinics.com**

patient-centered approach, while presenting widely varying scenarios for application of its principles.

Geoffrey P. Dunn, MD
Department of Surgery and
Palliative Care Consultation Service
UPMC Hamot Medical Center
2050 South Shore Drive
Erie, PA 16505, USA

E-mail address:
gpdunn1@earthlink.net

# Palliative Surgery in the Do-Not-Resuscitate Patient: Ethics and Practical Suggestions for Management

Thomas H. Scott, MD[a],*, Jonathan R. Gavrin, MD[b]

KEYWORDS

- Do-not-resuscitate • Palliative surgery
- Cardiopulmonary resuscitation • Self-determination

Much has changed in palliative care since 1999 when the senior author of this article published "Anesthesia and Palliative Care,"[1] in which he bemoaned the paucity of clinical and training programs, and encouraged anesthesiologists to get more involved. Not only has palliative care in the United States evolved into a well-recognized discipline of its own, with American Council for Graduate Medical Education (ACGME) subspecialty board certification and a rapidly growing number of dedicated fellowship slots, there also has been a concerted effort to educate the public, in addition to professionals, that palliative care is on the same continuum as standard care and demands aggressive symptom management, even when patients choose curative or life-prolonging therapies. Much of this push has been spearheaded by the Center to Advance Palliative Care (CAPC) (http://www.capc.org), a nonprofit organization that has worked tirelessly to promote the benefits of palliative care for alleviation of somatic and existential distress, as well the avoidance of unnecessary medical procedures and costs. The 1999 piece emphasized mostly common sense and compassionate ways in which anesthesiologists can contribute positively to the comfort of this vulnerable population. This article does not restate those points but rather focuses on the complexities and nuances of do-not-resuscitate (DNR) orders when patients present to the operating room (OR).

[a] Department of Anesthesiology and Critical Care, Perelman School of Medicine, University of Pennsylvania, Dulles 6, 3400 Spruce Street, Philadelphia, PA 19104, USA
[b] HUP Ethics Committee, Department of Anesthesiology and Critical Care, Hospital of the University of Pennsylvania, Dulles 6, 3400 Spruce Street, Philadelphia, PA 19104, USA
* Corresponding author.
*E-mail addresses:* Thomas.Scott2@uphs.upenn.edu; Thscott99@gmail.com

Anesthesiology Clin 30 (2012) 1–12
doi:10.1016/j.anclin.2012.02.001
1932-2275/12/$ – see front matter © 2012 Elsevier Inc. All rights reserved.

## CASE

*A 79-year-old woman with stage IV metastatic non–small cell lung cancer on hospice presents with increased hip pain. Her primary oncologist images the hip, and an impending hip fracture secondary to metastatic disease is diagnosed. She is offered an open reduction and internal fixation of her hip in the hopes of restoring some limited mobility and to provide pain relief at the end of her life so that she may attend her granddaughter's wedding. She is adamant that she not be resuscitated in the event of a cardiac arrest, and does not wish to be given vasopressors or to be intubated.*

Is it appropriate that the patient be allowed to maintain her DNR status during the perioperative period? Can hospice patients be taken to the OR for palliative surgery? Are her physicians required to honor her DNR decision in the OR? Is the surgeon or anesthesiologist obligated to provide care to a patient who refuses certain potentially lifesaving treatments? Are the patient and her family aware of the risk she is assuming by refusing resuscitation? Are there national guidelines that may help with the management of such a case?

Approximately 15% of patients with a DNR order will present for surgery.[2] The concept of a DNR order arises from the ethical principle of patient autonomy or self-determination. Just as a Jehovah's Witness may refuse blood transfusions, or a Christian Scientist may refuse to accept medical care, so too may any patient refuse any treatment for any reason. In ethics this is known as a "negative right" or right to refuse, and is always legitimate. Patient autonomy has limits, however. Although they may decline any therapy they choose, patients do not have the right to demand a treatment deemed medically inappropriate by their physician. There is no positive right, or right to demand on the part of patients.

Herein lies the challenge in palliative surgery: the patient's negative right to refuse treatment must be brought into balance with the physician's prerogative that he or she may refuse to provide any treatment deemed inconsistent with accepted standards of care. Specifically, interventions that are considered standard and necessary in the OR may be considered "resuscitation" on the hospital floor. Thus, if in the case outlined above the attending anesthesiologist considers that the only medically appropriate means of managing the patient's planned spinal anesthesia was with temporary use of vasopressors, the physician may negotiate with the patient for a transient suspension of her wish to have such vasopressors withheld. If she still refuses to accept vasopressors, the anesthesiologist would be within his rights to refuse to provide anesthesia for her case, as proceeding would not be consistent with accepted standards of care. This objection is a medical rather than a moral one, and is consistent with the physician's responsibility to provide only measures that are medically appropriate. With respect to moral objections (such as an anesthesiologist who objects to taking a DNR patient to OR on personal grounds), finding alternative staffing may be reasonable provided the case is nonemergent and alternative staffing can be arranged. Undue delay in palliative treatment owing to moral objections of perioperative staff is not appropriate. The fear of being treated differently and neglected may be a reason that patients elect to maintain their full-code status rather than waiving resuscitation.[3]

Were the patient taken to the OR and intubated or given vasopressors for any reason without a negotiated suspension of her explicit wish NOT to receive such treatments, this would constitute a violation of her right to self-determination and could be considered assault. Thus, before proceeding to the OR, a detailed discussion about the patient's goals and values in the context of the proposed surgery is mandatory on the part of both the surgeon and the anesthesiologist. Without such a conversation, there is a high risk of either violating a patient's right to self-determination, or the physician's right to refuse to proceed with a treatment that he or she feels is medically inappropriate. Current American Society of Anesthesiologists (ASA), American College of Surgeons (ACS), and Association of Perioperative Registered Nurses (AORN) guidelines all emphasize that it is an essential and required part of preoperative preparation for a patient with a standing DNR order to have and document a conversation regarding a patient's wishes with respect to limiting treatment during the perioperative period.[4–6]

## HISTORY OF DNR ORDERS IN THE PERIOPERATIVE PERIOD

Cardiopulmonary resuscitation (CPR) is the only medical intervention for which no consent is required, and an explicit physician's order is necessary for it to be withheld. Originally described as treatment for intraoperative cardiac arrest, its use has become widespread outside the OR and outside the hospital. Whereas mortality for intraoperative cardiac arrest was relatively low ($\sim$50%), survival figures for out-of-OR cardiac arrest were worse (10%–30%).[7,8]

Through the 1960s and 1970s as the practice of CPR disseminated, in the absence of professional or legal standards, physicians or hospital staff might decide who would be candidates for full resuscitation and who would not. This situation gave rise to the concept of a "slow code" or "Hollywood code," in which staff would proceed with less than full effort when the clinical situation was thought to be futile. Popular reaction to this practice was hostile, as patients and their families were sometimes left out of the decision to withhold CPR. In 1983 the President's Commission for the Study of Ethical Problems in Medicine clarified that, as a matter of national policy, patients had a right to expect CPR as the standard of care in all situations of cardiac arrest unless a patient's wish to have it withheld was clearly documented.[9] Since 1983, few people in the United States die in hospital without having CPR attempted.

Through the 1980s and up to 1991, another issue emerged. Patients' DNR orders were routinely rescinded on entering the OR.[10–13] There are numerous good reasons why this was thought to be reasonable. Many intraoperative cardiac arrests are a direct result of anesthesia or surgical complications, and can be corrected with an excellent clinical outcome. Moreover, physicians may be psychologically reluctant to take a patient into the OR if they feel unable to correct complications caused by their interventions. Measures that are standard in the OR and sometimes essential to a procedure's success might be considered resuscitation outside the OR. Clarifying these issues takes time. There may be little time to discuss the complexities and permutations of OR anesthesia and surgery with a busy OR schedule, especially when this conversation generally happens at the first meeting between the patient and the anesthesiologist. There was a perception that DNR patients would opt for a negotiated or conditional suspension of their DNR order when going to the OR after having a truly informed discussion about the implications of honoring a DNR in the OR.[11–14]

Anesthesiologists seem mostly to overlook the challenges of palliative surgery. Clemency and Thompson[10] showed in 1994 that anesthesiologists were twice as likely as either internists or surgeons to assume that DNR patients would suspend their DNR order in the OR. Anesthesiologists were also less likely to discuss the implications of a DNR order with their patients, less likely to refuse to provide care for a DNR patient, and more likely to ignore a patient's DNR request even if the patient made wishes explicit after an informed discussion. Thus, Robert Walker argued, patients presenting for palliative surgery "may be forced to weigh the benefits of [the] surgery against the risks of unwanted resuscitation."[13]

The routine suspension of a DNR order in the perioperative period (by policy or assumption) may be seen as consistent with the tradition of beneficence, promoting the well-being of patients and, perhaps, not exploring whether these practices violated certain patients' autonomy. Clarifying this issue, the Patient Self-Determination Act of 1990 (effective December 1991) established as United States law that a patient's right to self-determination was the supreme standard in medical ethics, taking precedence over beneficence.[15] Thus, several 1991 articles pointed out that routine suspension of DNR in the perioperative period violated a patient's right to self-determination.[11–14] In response, the ASA, the ACS, and AORN adopted guidelines in 1993-1994 supporting a "required reconsideration" of a patient's DNR status before proceeding with surgery.[4–6]

While well founded in principle, problems with implementation of required reconsideration were numerous. Standard advance directive forms, which resulted from the 1990 Patient Self-Determination Act, are mostly useless in clinical practice, being either vague (eg, "accept all treatment unless disease is incurable") or restrictive (eg, "no artificial life support"). Thus, patients often believe that they have a statement of their values and goals as a part of their advance directive, but in fact they do not. To properly inform a patient and "reconsider" the DNR status before palliative surgery, a long, exhaustive, and ideally multidisciplinary conversation with the patient, patient's surrogate decision maker, primary care physician, surgeon, and anesthesiologist must take place. Such a meeting is often impossible in clinical practice. Nonetheless, any conversation, even one that is not ideal, may suffice provided one addresses the patient's goals and values in the context of the procedure. This conversation should not ignore the patient's family unit as a whole and its understanding and acceptance of the possible outcomes of surgery. Nonsurrogate family members may not be decision makers, but they often have a deep emotional investment in the care of their loved one and should not be ignored. There are 4 possible results of required reconsideration: (1) maintain DNR status unaltered; (2) fully rescind DNR status in the perioperative period; (3) accept certain resuscitative measures but refuse others, which then must be documented fully; and (4) delegate to the anesthesiologist and/or surgeon the right to decide which interventions are appropriate and which are not pursuant to the patient's stated wishes.

ASA guidelines emphasize that this conversation is so important that it should not be delegated to another by the attending physician. The discussion should revolve around the patient's goals first, with those stated goals then applied to the procedure. In ethics this is known as a patient-regarding rather than a physician-regarding approach. In the aforementioned case the patient's stated goals are pain relief and attending her granddaughter's wedding. With respect to the procedure, if she does not wish to be intubated then a neuraxial technique would be required. Thus, discussion may then relate to the role of vasopressors in the perioperative period with neuraxial anesthesia. Clinical care must focus on the patient's goals and values, not on clinical outcomes. Consequently, iatrogenic death directly attributable to anesthetic or surgical complications may be appropriate and acceptable as long as care is consistent with accepted standards of practice. In other words, if the patient insists that she would accept neither vasopressors nor intubation, many anesthesiologists may consider this medically inappropriate. This would be a medical, rather than a moral, objection. If, however, she accepts vasopressors but would not accept closed-chest compressions or intubation under any circumstances, then, should she experience a cardiac arrest (such as asystole directly attributable to her spinal anesthesia), she would expire and such a death should be recorded as "expected" in any hospital morbidity statistics. Again, the important point is not assuring a particular outcome, but rather ensuring that care is designed around the patient's individual goals and values, and is medically consistent with standards of care.

Because the purpose of the DNR order and advanced directives is to give patients the right to self-determination with respect to their care at the end of life, some have voiced concerns that allowing a physician to act as a surrogate decision maker may place too much authority back in the hands of physicians.[16] Indeed, it is difficult to fathom how an anesthesiologist, usually meeting a patient for the first time just before surgery, would be in a position to truly understand a patient's goals and values well enough to act as the proxy intraoperatively. That said, in contrast to previous decades when patients were excluded from the decision as to what kinds of resuscitations they would be offered, giving the patient the option of making the anesthesiologist or surgeon the surrogate decision maker still respects patient autonomy and is not inappropriate.[17] Current ASA guidelines explicitly state "The patient or designated surrogate may allow the anesthesiologist and surgical team to use clinical judgment in determining which resuscitation procedures are appropriate in the context of the situation and the patient's stated goals and values."[4] Where possible, however, it would be advisable to consult with a clearly identified nonphysician surrogate decision maker for guidance in the rare event of an ongoing resuscitation in an incapacitated patient.

## HOSPICE PATIENTS

There is a common misunderstanding that patients who have enrolled in hospice also have given up the desire for resuscitation. Designating oneself as DNR is not necessary for hospice care. Only 2 requirements must be met for someone to be eligible for hospice: (a) the patient, or designated surrogate, expressly desires to focus on comfort and quality of life, while forgoing curative therapies for the primary, life-threatening disease; and (b) a physician certifies that the patient has a life expectancy of 6 months or less, if the illness runs its natural course.

No one ever gives up the right to palliation, including surgery, if the interventions are consistent with patient goals, values, and comfort. Hospice benefits may be renewed for as long as needed, if the illness does not "run its natural course." A patient may disenroll from hospice at any time.

In addition, patients may continue to obtain treatment for conditions not related to the illness that qualified them for hospice, including surgical interventions. If, for instance, a hospice enrollee with metastatic lung cancer develops an acute appendicitis, incarcerated hernia, or any other condition amenable to surgical intervention, he or she should receive the same care as would a nonhospice patient. In such cases, a DNR order may exist for which the same principles discussed in this article will apply.

## SUGGESTED PRACTICAL APPROACH TO THE PREOPERATIVE EVALUATION OF THE DNR PATIENT PRESENTING FOR SURGERY

- Uniform policies suspending DNR orders before surgery are inappropriate and are not useful.
- It is essential and required that a discussion with the patient regarding values and goals take place and that those values and goals be discussed in the context of the specific procedure and anesthesia required.

**Table 1**
Treatment of somatic distress and side effects of medication

| Cause of Distress | Comfort Care Modalities | Mechanism of Action | Major Side Effects | Relief of Side Effects |
|---|---|---|---|---|
| Pain | Acetaminophen | Analgesic, antipyretic | None except with overdose | N/A |
| | Aspirin and NSAIDs | Analgesic, antipyretic Anti-inflammatory | GI upset & ulceration Platelet dysfunction | Antacids, sucralfate, omeprazole, $H_2$ blockers, omeprazole, misoprostol |
| | Opioids | Analgesic | Nausea | Antiemetics |
| | | | Constipation | Laxatives, stool softeners |
| | | | Sedation | Reduce dose, stimulants |
| | | | Pruritus | Antihistamines, nalbuphine, naloxone |
| | | | Urinary retention | Reduce dose, catheterize Nalbuphine (?), naloxone |
| Nausea/emesis | Scopolamine | Anticholinergic | Dry mouth, confusion | Reduce dose or discontinue |
| | Dimenhydrinate | Anticholinergic, antihistamine | Confusion, dry mouth | Reduce dose or discontinue |
| | Diphenhydramine | Antihistamine | Sedation, dry mouth, Confusion | Reduce dose or discontinue |
| | Promethazine | Antihistamine | Sedation, dry mouth, confusion | Reduce dose or discontinue |
| | Hydroxyzine | Antihistamine | Sedation, dry mouth, confusion | Reduce dose or discontinue |
| | Ondansetron Granisetron | Antiserotonin (5HT-3) | Headache | Analgesics Discontinue |
| | Haloperidol Droperidol | Antidopamine | Extrapyramidal symptoms, sedation | Diphenhydramine, cogentin Reduce dose or discontinue |
| | Phenothiazines (not promethazine) | Antidopamine | Extrapyramidal symptoms, sedation | Diphenhydramine, cogentin Reduce dose or discontinue |
| | Metoclopramide | Antidopamine Gastric emptying | Extrapyramidal symptoms, sedation | Diphenhydramine, cogentin Reduce dose or discontinue |

| | Drug | Mechanism | Side effects | Recommendation |
|---|---|---|---|---|
| | benzodiazepines | Unknown (?) Effect on limbic system | Sedation, depression, confusion | Reduce dose or discontinue |
| | Cannabinoids | CB(1) agonist (?) Effect on limbic system | Sedation, confusion | Reduce dose or discontinue |
| | Corticosteroids | Unknown | Confusion, sleep disruption | Haloperidol may help |
| | Aprepitant | Substance P antagonist | Fatigue, constipation, diarrhea | Activating drugs, GI medication |
| | Olanzapine | Antidopamine Antiserotonin (5HT-2) | Variety, including extrapyramidal symptoms | Discontinue drug |
| Dyspnea | β-Agonists | Bronchodilation | Tachycardia, restlessness | Sedative |
| | Anticholinergics | Bronchodilation | Tachycardia, dry mouth | |
| | Methylxanthines | Bronchodilation, (?) Increased strength | Tachycardia, CNS symptoms with overdose | Decrease dose |
| | Opioids | Shift $CO_2$ response, sedation | Tachycardia, CNS symptoms with overdose | Decrease dose |
| | Benzodiazepines | Shift $CO_2$ response, anxiolysis, sedation | Tachycardia, CNS symptoms with overdose | Decrease dose |
| | Alcohol | Anxiolysis, sedation | Oversedation, confusion | Reduce dose or discontinue |
| | Barbiturates | Shift $CO_2$ response, anxiolysis, sedation | Oversedation, memory loss | Reduce dose or discontinue |
| Cough | Potassium iodide | Pharyngeal lubrication | Potassium toxicity | Discontinue drug |
| | Opioids | Antitussive | Potassium toxicity | Discontinue drug |
| Sedation | Methylphenidate | CNS stimulant | Agitation | Discontinue drug |
| | Amphetamines | CNS stimulant | Agitation, tachyphylaxis | Discontinue drug |
| | Modafinil | Wakefulness promoter | Headache, anxiety, insomnia | Discontinue drug |

Abbreviations: CNS, central nervous system; GI, gastrointestinal; N/A, no data available; NSAID, nonsteroidal anti-inflammatory drug.

**Table 2**
**Equianalgesic doses and common starting doses**

| Opioid | Equianalgesic Parenteral Dose (mg) | Equianalgesic PO Dose (mg) | Starting Dose Adults (>50 kg) | Starting Dose Children (<50 kg) |
|---|---|---|---|---|
| Morphine | 10 | 30–60[a] | 15 mg PO | 0.05–0.1 mg/kg IV |
| Meperidine | 75 | 300 | 12.5 mg[b] or 100 mg IV | 1 mg/kg (maximum 100 mg/dose) |
| Hydromorphone | 1.5 | 4–6 | 2–6 mg PO | 0.015 mg/kg IV |
| Fentanyl | 0.1 | N/A | 0.5–2 µg/kg IV | 1–10 µg/kg |
| Sufentanil | 0.01[c] | N/A | 0.5–2 µg/kg IV[d] | 0.1–5 µg/kg[d] |
| Alfentanil | 1[c] | N/A | 50–150 µg/kg IV[d] | 5–50 µg/kg[e] |
| Remifentanil | 0.1[c] | N/A | 1–4 µg/kg[d] | 0.4–1 µg/kg[f]; 0.25–1 µg/kg[g] |
| Codeine | 120 | 200 | 30–60 mg PO | 0.5–1.0 mg/kg (2–6 y old) |
| Hydrocodone | N/A | 20–30 | 5 mg PO | 0.125 mg/kg |
| Oxycodone | N/A | 20–40 | 5–20 mg PO | 0.1 mg/kg |
| Tramadol | 100[h] | 300–600 | 25–50 mg PO | Not established in children |
| Methadone | 2.0 | 6.7, 1[i] | 2.5–5 mg PO | 0.1–0.2 mg/kg every 6 h, maximum 10 mg/dose |
| Nalbuphine | N/A | N/A | 10 mg IV | 0.05–0.1 mg/kg |

Because of incomplete cross-tolerance and significant variation in pharmacodynamics between individuals, extreme caution must be exercised when converting from one opioid to another. The equianalgesic values presented here are approximate and intended to demonstrate relative potency and not necessarily clinically precise opioid conversion values (eg, the methadone value is only for converting from methadone to morphine, NOT vice versa).

[a] 30 mg for chronic dosing, 60 mg for acute dosing.

[b] 12.5 mg dose is for treating postoperative or amphotericin-associated shivering, 100 mg for mild to moderate pain.

[c] Relative potency based on amount required to reduce the minimal alveolar concentration of isoflurane by 50%.

[d] Infusion rates and loading doses vary depending on whether the goal is sedation, analgesia, or anesthesia. Loading doses should be given gradually, over 2 to 5 minutes. Boluses are often associated with apnea and chest wall rigidity. Infusion rates for sufentanil, alfentanil, and remifentanil, depending on nature and duration of surgery, are 0.1 to 1 µg/kg/h, 0.5 to 3 µg/kg/min, and 0.1 to 0.4 µg/kg/min, respectively. In children and infants, sufentanil may be used for sedation or anesthesia (usually cardiac). For sedation of children in the intensive care unit, a bolus of 0.1 to 0.5 µg/kg followed by infusion of 0.005 to 0.01 µg/kg/min, or for anesthesia (usually cardiac) a bolus of 1 to 5 µg/kg followed by 0.01 to 0.05 µg/kg/min should be administered.

[e] Average dose needed for sedation in infants and neonates about 20 µg/kg.

[f] Dose for infants from birth to 1 year old.

[g] Dose for children 1 to 12 years old.

[h] Intravenous form not available in the United States.

[i] Converting from methadone to another opioid is complicated and should only be attempted by clinicians familiar with its use. 6.7 mg should be used for acute dose conversion, 1 mg should be used for chronic dose conversion from methadone to morphine.

*Data from* Refs.[19–30]

- ○ This discussion should be undertaken by the attending physician and not delegated.
- ○ If resuscitation is to be limited, the patient may choose to appoint the anesthesiologist or surgeon as a surrogate decision maker in the OR. The physician surrogate agrees that any decisions regarding resuscitation will, to the best of his or her knowledge, reflect the patient's stated values and goals in the context of the procedure. This should be documented in the chart.
- ○ If the patient does not wish to make the anesthesiologist or surgeon the surrogate, then the patient must list which specific therapies and interventions would be acceptable and which would be refused. Unfortunately, this can be a cumbersome, but necessary, process.
- ○ If a negotiated suspension of the patient's DNR status is agreed to, then the precise time or location when the perioperative period ends should be specified in the chart.
- ○ Whenever possible, this discussion should be multidisciplinary and include the patient's primary care physician, surgeon, and anesthesiologist, as well as his or her surrogate decision maker.
- ○ Whenever possible, the patient's family should be aware of the results of this conversation and express understanding of its implications.
- Whenever possible, a nonphysician surrogate decision maker should be identified preoperatively and be available at all times throughout the perioperative period.
- Physicians may object to patients' stated goals and directives on 2 grounds:
  - ○ Medical objection. A patient is refusing a specific therapy such that proceeding with the intervention would not be consistent with accepted standards of care or, in the judgment of the physician, compromises safety. Medical objections are a reasonable justification for delaying an intervention.
    - Conflicts of this type should be handled by an appropriate institutional body, usually an ethics consultation.
  - ○ Personal or moral objection. If the anesthesiologist or surgeon has personal or moral objections to the patient's views, that practitioner should withdraw from the case in a nonjudgmental fashion, provided alternative staffing can be arranged.
    - If alternative staffing is not readily available, it is not acceptable to delay palliative surgery based on one's own personal objections.

## INTRAOPERATIVE AND POSTOPERATIVE SYMPTOM MANAGEMENT

The anesthesiologist is in a unique position to alleviate suffering. Focus should be not only on providing adequate analgesia but also on other common symptoms more common in the palliative care population: dyspnea, cough, sedation, anxiety, and nausea. In addition, the DNR patient may be older, sicker, and require larger doses of opioids, increasing the risk of postoperative delirium.[18] Appropriate treatment of symptoms while minimizing the risk of complications is, of course, precisely the day-to-day routine of all perioperative physicians. A detailed discussion of how this is done is beyond the scope of this article. **Table 1** summarizes various palliative medical therapies, their indications, and likely side effects, and **Table 2**[19–30] provides approximate ratios of opioid equianalgesic conversion ratios. Opioid conversions should always be undertaken cautiously, as incomplete cross-tolerance and enormous variation between individual responses can result in inadequate analgesia or opioid-induced hypotension, somnolence, and apnea.

## SUMMARY

Whereas palliative care in the United States was in its relative infancy just a decade ago, it has made tremendous strides in the intervening years. The central tenets of providing symptom management and comfort for all patients, no matter what the stage of their illness, and to address goals of care and personal values in the context of the patient-family unit, are widespread now. These tenets are consistent with the burgeoning movement toward patient- and family-centered care, away from practitioner- and institution-centered practices. One of the most perplexing issues arises when a palliative care patient presents to the OR with an already existing DNR order. This article describes the most common conflicting issues that may arise and provides guidance to surgeons, anesthesiologists, patients, and their primary physicians in reaching satisfactory resolution and optimal care of the patient. In keeping with the published ASA guidelines, the authors believe that anesthesia departments should appoint a liaison to the surgery and perioperative nursing departments to provide education and create an atmosphere conducive to discussions with palliative care patients about goals of care, including DNR status. Whenever time permits, these discussions should include everyone important to the patient's care, from preparation to the postoperative period.

## REFERENCES

1. Gavrin J. Anesthesiology and palliative care. Anesthesiol Clin North Am 1999;17: 467–77.
2. La Puma J, Silverstein MD, Stocking CB, et al. Life-sustaining treatment. A prospective study of patients with DNR orders in a teaching hospital. Arch Intern Med 1988;148(10):2193–8. Available at: http://elinks.library.upenn.edu/sfx_local? sid=OVID:medline&id=pmid:3178377. Accessed January 29, 2012.
3. Ewanchuk M, Brindley PG. Perioperative do-not-resuscitate orders—doing 'nothing' when 'something' can be done. Crit Care 2006;10(4):219. Available at: http://ovidsp.ovid.com/ovidweb.cgi?T=JS&CSC=Y&NEWS=N&PAGE=fulltext& D=med4&AN=16834763; http://elinks.library.upenn.edu/sfx_local?sid=OVID: medline&id=pmid:16834763. Accessed January 29, 2012.
4. American Society of Anesthesiologists. Ethical guidelines for the anesthesia care of patients with do-not-resuscitate orders or other directives that limit treatment. Available at: http://www.asahq.org/For-Members/~/media/For%20Members/ documents/Standards%20Guidelines%20Stmts/Ethical%20Guidelines%20for%20 the%20Anesthesia%20Care%20of%20Patients.ashx. Accessed January 29, 2012.
5. American College of Surgeons. Statement on advance directives by patients: "Do not resuscitate" in the operating room. Bull Am Coll Surg 1994;94:29.
6. American Association of Perioperative Nurses (AORN). Perioperative care of patients with do-not-resuscitate or allow-natural-death orders. Available at: http://www.aorn.org/WorkArea/DownloadAsset.aspx?id=219172012. Accessed January 29, 2012.
7. Deasy C, Bray JE, Smith K, et al. Cardiac arrest outcomes before and after the 2005 resuscitation guidelines implementation: evidence of improvement? Resuscitation 2011;82(8):984–8. Available at: http://ovidsp.ovid.com/ovidweb.cgi? T=JS&CSC=Y&NEWS=N&PAGE=fulltext&D=medl&AN=21536367; http://elinks. library.upenn.edu/sfx_local?sid=OVID:medline&id=pmid:21536367. Accessed January 29, 2012.
8. Sprung J, Warner ME, Contreras MG, et al. Predictors of survival following cardiac arrest in patients undergoing noncardiac surgery: a study of 518,294 patients at

a tertiary referral center. Anesthesiology 2003;99(2):259–69. Available at: http://ovidsp.ovid.com/ovidweb.cgi?T=JS&CSC=Y&NEWS=N&PAGE=fulltext&D=med4&AN=12883397; http://elinks.library.upenn.edu/sfx_local?sid=OVID:medline&id=pmid:12883397. Accessed January 29, 2012.

9. President's Commission for the Study of Ethical Problems in Medicine and Biomedical and Behavioral Research. Deciding to forego life-sustaining treatment: ethical, medical, and legal issues in treatment decisions. Library of Congress; 1983. 83-600503. p. 1–554.

10. Clemency MV, Thompson NJ. "Do not resuscitate" (DNR) orders in the perioperative period—a comparison of the perspectives of anesthesiologists, internists, and surgeons. Anesth Analg 1994;78(4):651–8. Available at: http://elinks.library.upenn.edu/sfx_local?sid=OVID:medline&id=pmid:8135382. Accessed January 29, 2012.

11. Cohen CB, Cohen PJ. Do-not-resuscitate orders in the operating room. N Engl J Med 1991;325(26):1879–82. Available at: http://elinks.library.upenn.edu/sfx_local?sid=OVID:medline&id=pmid:1961228. Accessed January 29, 2012.

12. Truog RD. "Do-not-resuscitate" orders during anesthesia and surgery. Anesthesiology 1991;74(3):606–8. Available at: http://ovidsp.ovid.com/ovidweb.cgi?T=JS&CSC=Y&NEWS=N&PAGE=fulltext&D=med3&AN=2001038; http://elinks.library.upenn.edu/sfx_local?sid=OVID:medline&id=pmid:2001038. Accessed January 29, 2012.

13. Walker RM. DNR in the OR. resuscitation as an operative risk. JAMA 1991;266(17):2407–12. Available at: http://elinks.library.upenn.edu/sfx_local?sid=OVID:medline&id=pmid:1717723. Accessed January 29, 2012.

14. Martin RL, Soifer BE, Stevens WC. Ethical issues in anesthesia: management of the do-not-resuscitate patient. Anesth Analg 1991;73(2):221–5. Available at: http://elinks.library.upenn.edu/sfx_local?sid=OVID:medline&id=pmid:1854037. Accessed January 29, 2012.

15. Panetta L. Omnibus budget reconciliation act of 1990. United States House of Representatives. 1990.

16. Jackson SH, Van Norman GA. Goals- and values-directed approach to informed consent in the "DNR" patient presenting for surgery: more demanding of the anesthesiologist? Anesthesiology 1999;90(1):3–6. Available at: http://elinks.library.upenn.edu/sfx_local?sid=OVID:medline&id=pmid:9915306. Accessed January 29, 2012.

17. Truog RD, Waisel DB, Burns JP. DNR in the OR: a goal-directed approach. Anesthesiology 1999;90(1):289–95. Available at: http://ovidsp.ovid.com/ovidweb.cgi?T=JS&CSC=Y&NEWS=N&PAGE=fulltext&D=med4&AN=9915337; http://elinks.library.upenn.edu/sfx_local?sid=OVID:medline&id=pmid:9915337. Accessed January 29, 2012.

18. Pisani MA, Murphy TE, Araujo KL, et al. Factors associated with persistent delirium after intensive care unit admission in an older medical patient population. J Crit Care 2010;25(3):540, e1–7. Available at: http://ovidsp.ovid.com/ovidweb.cgi?T=JS&CSC=Y&NEWS=N&PAGE=fulltext&D=medl&AN=20413252; http://elinks.library.upenn.edu/sfx_local?sid=OVID:medline&id=pmid:20413252. Accessed January 29, 2012.

19. Micromedex. Available at: http://proxy.library.upenn.edu:2135/hcs/librarian. Accessed December 15, 2010.

20. Available at: http://www.PDR.net; http://www.pdr.net/Default.aspx. Accessed December 15, 2010.

21. Daily Med. Available at: http://dailymed.nlm.nih.gov/dailymed/about.cfm. Accessed December 15, 2010.

22. Hydromorphone Hydrochloride [Package Insert]. Available at: http://pharmaceuticals.covidien.com/imageServer.aspx/doc192059.pdf?contentID=16008&contenttype=application/pdf. Accessed December 15, 2010.
23. Chhabra S, Bull J. Methadone. Am J Hosp Palliat Care 2008;25(2):146–50.
24. Fukuda K. Intravenous opioid anesthetics. In: Miller RD, editor. Miller's anesthesia. 6th edition. Philadelphia: Elsevier Churchill Livingstone; 2005. p. 379–423. Chapter 11.
25. Inturrisi CE. Opioid analgesics. In: Ballantyne J, Fishman S, Rathmell JP, editors. Bonica's management of pain. 4th edition. Baltimore (MD): Lippincott, Williams, and Wilkins; 2010. p. 1172–87. Chapter 78.
26. Kalso E. Oxycodone. J Pain Symptom Manage 2005;29(Suppl 5):S47–56.
27. Rosow C, Dershwitz M. Pharmacology of opioid analgesics. In: Longnecker DE, Brown DL, Newman MF, et al, editors. Anesthesiology. 1st edition. China: McGraw Hill; 2008. p. 869–96. Chapter 41.
28. Stein C, Hug CC. Opioids in pain control: basic and clinical aspects. Cambridge (UK): Cambridge University Press; 1999.
29. Thompson JE. A practical guide to contemporary pharmacy practice (Point (Lippincott Williams & Wilkins)). 3rd edition. Philadelphia (PA): Lippincott Williams & Wilkins; 2009.
30. Trescot AM, Datta S, Lee M, et al. Opioid pharmacology. Pain Physician 2008; 11(Suppl 2):S133–53.

# Surgical Palliative Care: Recent Trends and Developments

Geoffrey P. Dunn, MD

## KEYWORDS

- Palliative care • Surgical palliative care • Palliative surgery
- Symptom management • End-of-life care

## VIGNETTES: THEN AND NOW
### 1985

A 55-year-old woman with a history of stage III ovarian carcinoma, 1 year after total abdominal hysterectomy, bilateral salpingo-oophorectomy and omentectomy, and several cycles of cisplatin-based chemotherapy, presents at a 350-bed regional medical center with increasing abdominal pain and distention, nausea, and vomiting. She was told she was stable at her last outpatient oncology evaluation 2 months previously when she was complaining of abdominal pain, numbness in her feet, and loss of appetite. She is receiving no regular medications except propoxyphene with acetaminophen (Darvocet) as needed for abdominal pain. On physical examination she is pale and cachectic. She has diminished breath sounds with dullness to percussion at each lung base, more so on the right. Her abdomen is distended with a remote midline incision.

Bowel sounds are high pitched. She has shifting dullness to percussion and multiple palpable abdominal masses. She has no guarding. Plain abdominal radiographs are consistent with a small-bowel obstruction. Bilateral moderate-sized pleural effusions are noted on the chest radiograph. The surgeon tells her he thinks she has a bowel obstruction from her cancer and he would like to avoid operating if at all possible. A nasogastric (NG) tube is inserted and placed to continuous suction. She is not given opioid analgesia because of the surgeon's fear of masking peritoneal signs. After 5 days of nonoperative therapy the patient is advised that her condition mandates surgery because of persistent obstruction and fears of potential gangrenous bowel. She signs an operative consent for exploratory laparotomy, possible bowel resection, removal of tumor, possible formation of ostomy, and insertion of central venous catheter. Potential complications listed include failure to remove the entire tumor,

---

A version of this article was published in the 91:2 issue of *Surgical Clinics of North America*.
The author has nothing to disclose.
Department of Surgery and Palliative Care Consultation Service, UPMC Hamot Medical Center, 2050 South Shore Drive, Erie, PA 16505, USA
*E-mail address:* gpdunn1@earthlink.net

reobstruction, bleeding, bowel injury, wound hernia, fistula formation, and pneumo-thorax. The patient confides to her nurse that she is worried the surgeon, "will not be able to remove all of the tumor." The patient proceeds to an exploratory laparotomy by an experienced general surgeon assisted by a third-year surgical resident. While at the scrub sink, the surgeon tells the resident, "This will probably be an exercise in futility. I feel like an executioner. At least this way, she might not live the rest of her life with an NG tube stuck down her nose." After making a generous midline incision, a large amount of ascites and multiple points of small-bowel obstruction secondary to bulky tumor are noted. Additionally, extensive studding of all peritoneal surfaces with tumor is noted. A gastrostomy for drainage is placed and subclavian venous access is established for administration of total parenteral nutrition. The surgeon discloses the findings to the patient's husband in a busy waiting room. "Unfortunately, there was nothing we could do but palliate her with a gastrostomy tube. We will see what the oncologists can recommend and give her intravenous nutrition so she will not starve." The following day, the same findings are disclosed to the patient in the same fashion as disclosed to her husband by the surgeon during morning rounds. The patient asks, "What happens next?" to which the surgeon responds, "It's in God's hands at this point." The patient's postoperative analgesia orders specify meperidine 25 to 50 mg intramuscularly (IM) every 3 hours as needed and hydroxyzine 25 mg IM every 3 hours as needed. The consulting oncologist tells the patient he would like to defer chemo-therapy until the patient "becomes stronger." A close friend of the patient privately asks the surgeon, "what he knows about hospice," to which he scornfully responds, "What are they going to do for her, kill her with morphine?" On the fourth postoperative day, bilious drainage begins draining from the midline incision at the site of an external retention suture, which necessitates placement of an ostomy drainage bag. Two days later, the patient becomes lethargic, hypotensive, and anuric and is transferred to the surgical intensive care unit (SICU). Because of the hypotension, her nurse withholds her pain medication but exhorts her to "not give up." Because of ongoing hypotension and hypoxemia, an arterial line and Swan-Ganz catheter are inserted, vasopressor support is initiated, and the patient is intubated for ventilator support. She receives multiple infusions of albumin and frequent boluses of crystalloid. A right-sided thora-costomy tube is placed because of an increasingly large pleural effusion. After 2 days, the patient becomes increasingly obtunded and hypotensive, and then develops ventricular ectopy, which is followed by ventricular fibrillation. She is defibrillated but is unable to resume a cardiac rhythm and is pronounced dead by the ICU resident. The family is notified by telephone and asked to come to the hospital for her personal effects. One week later her case is presented at the surgical department's mortality and morbidity rounds because of her postoperative complication and death. The consensus of the surgeons present is "What else could you [the surgeon] do?"

## 2010

A 55-year-old woman with a history of stage III ovarian carcinoma, 3 years status after total abdominal hysterectomy, bilateral salpingo-oophorectomy and omentectomy, and subsequent carboplatin, paclitaxel, and topotecan chemotherapy presents at a 350-bed regional medical center with increasing abdominal distention, abdominal pain, nausea, and vomiting. Further questioning reveals she has dyspnea and profound weakness. She is an active member of an ovarian cancer support group facilitated by a health care professional. A palliative care team at the outpatient cancer treatment center actively follows her for management of her cancer-related pain and chemotherapy-induced neuropathic pain. She is receiving 160 mg extended-release morphine daily, with 20 mg immediate-release morphine every 2 hours as needed for breakthrough pain and gabapentin 600 mg daily for her neuropathic pain. Additionally, she is taking megestrol acetate 600 mg daily for appetite stimulation and mirtazapine15 mg daily for depression and sleeplessness.

At the time of her admission, her surgeon assesses her pain during which she reports generalized abdominal pain with an intensity of 8 to 9 out of 10 with pain spikes "above 10." Her pain was well controlled 1 week previously. On physical examination she is pale and cachectic. She has diminished breath sounds with dullness to percussion at each lung base, more so on the right. Her abdomen is distended with a remote midline incision.

Bowel sounds are high pitched. She has shifting dullness to percussion and multiple palpable abdominal masses. She has no guarding. The surgeon explains to the patient that he would like to make her more comfortable before initiating any diagnostics or conversation to which she promptly agrees. He orders morphine 20 mg intravenously (IV) every 4 hours with 10 mg IV every 2 hours as needed for breakthrough pain. Following this, a nasogastric tube is inserted and two liters of bilious fluid is drained.

The surgeon explains to her that he will now order a CT scan of the abdomen and pelvis with contrast to determine the site of obstruction, its probable cause, and extent of her disease. He asks her to invite others of her choosing to be present later when he discusses the results in her room. He states that he is concerned that among the possible reasons for her clinical presentation is progressing disease, in which case several important decisions will have to be made. The patient indicates she will have her husband present. CT of the abdomen and pelvis shows evidence of small-bowel obstruction, a small amount of ascites, and disseminated bulky disease. She also is noted to have a large right pleural effusion. Laboratory results include prealbumin (7 mg/dL), hematocrit (23%), and CA 125 (7000 U/mL). The surgeon asks the patient's nurse to accompany him during his meeting with the patient and her husband. He turns off his beeper, introduces himself to the patient's husband and sits down in a chair next to the patient. After he determines that her pain is now well controlled ("2 out of 10, much better"), the surgeon asks them what they already know about her illness and if they are willing to hear any new important information. Both indicate their willingness to proceed with the discussion. The patient says, "I know it isn't looking good, my oncologist said we have about run out of options. My CA 125 has been going up but I am hoping it's the chemo that has been making me so weak and sick. My support group has been telling me to seek another opinion. I don't want to give up for my family's sake," looking pleadingly at her husband, "but I don't think I can do this anymore." The surgeon acknowledges how difficult this must be with her physical discomfort and her concerns for her family. The husband speaks up and says, tearfully, "I just don't want her to suffer." The surgeon acknowledges that he can see that this is his wish. He then tells them that the scan and blood tests have confirmed their fears, that the cancer has significantly progressed and has now caused a bowel blockage. He tells them there is also a large amount of fluid in the right chest cavity. The surgeon remains silent as she reacts to the news with a knowing downward look nodding her head and crying softly. He offers her a tissue and states, "I can see this has come as a sad disappointment to you," turning to the husband, "and you." After a long period of silence she states, "what next?" The husband asks if surgery can relieve her blockage. The surgeon says, "Let's go back to what you said about your wish that she not suffer and use that as the standard by which we decide what to do and what not do. Surgery is theoretically possible, although I am not recommending it for several reasons. She has some of the features that predict poor survival and quality-of-life outcomes from surgery in this situation: the fluid in her abdomen; the multiple bulky masses; and most importantly, the failure of multiple chemotherapy regimens to control the disease. Additionally, she has poor nutritional status, and, as she has said she is tired, in the sense that her reserves are exhausted. Even if surgery relieved her blockage, it will not restore her strength or appetite." The patient's husband looks bewildered and states, "What do you do if you don't operate and she can't eat?" The surgeon responds, "Let me break this down into several answers because there are several forms of discomfort or suffering her illness can cause. We can relieve her of the symptoms of bowel obstruction and the fluid in her abdomen and chest cavities using a combination of medications and procedures less invasive than an open operation. While this is getting underway, we will work on preparing for your ongoing support after she is out of the hospital. Your question about eating is more of a challenge because we equate eating with health and survival and food is such a central part of the way we relate to others. The lack of appetite and the ability for the body to turn nutrients into beneficial protein is a part of her illness. It's not lack of food that is making her ill, it's her illness that is now making the benefit of food impossible, which is not starving in the usual sense of the word. The word *starving* implies that the restoration of lacking nutrients would reverse the condition. That is, unfortunately, not the case here." The surgeon continues, looking at the husband, "You may be less distressed to know that she is probably indifferent to food and would be relieved to not have it be the focus at this point." The patient nods affirmatively. The surgeon concludes by explaining the regimen of medications he will use to give her relief from her bowel obstruction, explaining that she may have an occasional emesis but that is generally acceptable to patients if their nausea and pain are controlled. He then tells her he will be in again later to see if she is getting relief and to answer further questions. In addition to the morphine she is receiving, he orders octreotide 250 μg subcutaneously every 12 hours and prochlorperazine 10 mg IV every 6 hours, and then removes her nasogastric tube. When he returns several hours later she is comfortable. She tells the surgeon, "I want to go home." The surgeon confirms with them that they have accepted his recommendation not to have surgery and instead focus on keeping her comfortable and expediting her return home. He states that he is confident that she can be kept comfortable in her home setting with the proper support. She then asks him, "How long can this go?" The surgeon asks the patient and her husband if they are ready to discuss prognosis at this time, to which they both respond definitely yes. The surgeon says, "When we give estimates, we are giving averages of all patients with similar problems, not necessarily what will happen to you. Our best way of making an estimate is the change in the person's functional status, in other words, what you are able to do during a day. If you are bedbound and with a known progressive, life-limiting illness such as yours and requiring total care, survival is measured in weeks or less." Silence follows. The surgeon tells them, "I can see how sad this is making you." The patient says, "Actually, that is what I figured. When can I go?" The surgeon responds by telling them she could leave as soon as her home is ready and her symptoms are reliably controlled. He tells them that the best support available to fulfill her wish to be home and keep her symptoms controlled would be a hospice program. The surgeon tells them it would be prudent to clarify at this time her future preferences for interventions, such as cardiopulmonary resuscitation, ventilator support, intravenous hydration, and artificial nutrition. The patient says she is no longer interested in these interventions, to which the surgeon responds that he supports her preferences because of the marginal benefit these interventions would bestow during this phase of her illness. He asks them if they think they have the spiritual support they would want at this time, to which they respond they have already met with their pastor earlier in the day. Although her medication is controlling her symptoms well, the patient elects an endoscopic percutaneous gastrostomy (PEG) insertion for drainage. Additionally, the right pleural effusion is drained under CT guidance. Arrangements with a home hospice agency are subsequently made and she returns home the day following PEG placement. Her symptoms remain controlled at home and she is even able to eat small amounts of low-residue food. She succumbs 10 days later, peacefully, surrounded by her family. Several days later, during calling hours before her funeral, the patient's husband gives the surgeon a long silent hug when the surgeon greets him. He says to the surgeon, "You could not have done more for me and my wife."

Palliation has been an essential, if not the primary, activity of surgery during much of its history. However, it has been only during the past decade that the modern principles and practices of palliative care, which were developed in nonsurgical specialties in the United States and abroad, have been introduced to surgical institutions, widely varied practice settings, education, and research. Because of its relevance to surgery, the specialty of anesthesia will inevitably be influenced by these developments as well. The Ether Monument in the Boston Public Garden, erected by a citizen grateful for the contribution of anesthesia to the relief of human suffering, reminds us that the specialty of anesthesia, like that of surgery, is rooted in the impulse to relieve suffering, something that may be overlooked in an era of increased focus on physiologic monitoring and perioperative risk reduction.

The experience and success of the hospice movement in the United States and abroad undoubtedly has facilitated the acceptance and development of the field of palliative medicine, although not without some resistance from all medical specialties and the public because of hospice's association with the dying process and the persistence of a death-denying popular and medical culture. The conceptual and psychological challenge for surgeons is the assimilation of principles (patient/family unit as the unit of care, relief of suffering, spiritual growth) first learned from hospice care, which were subsequently adapted to the much larger population of patients with advanced, but not necessarily terminal, illness. This reframing of the goal of care requires a shift from the biophysical (disease-focused) model to a model centered upon suffering or existential considerations independent of the treatment's impact upon the disease processes.

Palliative care is interdisciplinary care that aims to relieve suffering and improve quality of life for patients and their families in the context of serious illness. It is offered simultaneously with all other appropriate medical treatment and its indication is not limited to situations associated with a poor prognosis for survival. Palliative care strives to achieve more than symptom control, but it should not be confused with noncurative treatment. Palliative care is not the opposite of curative treatment. Noncurative treatment is the opposite of curative treatment. *Surgical* palliative care is the treatment of suffering and the promotion of quality of life for patients who are seriously or terminally ill under surgical care (**Table 1**).[1]

The previous strongly contrasting vignettes, taken directly from the author's clinical experience, demonstrate the impact of the growing field of palliative care on surgical practice. Many of the interventions; communication approaches; and the scientific, ethical, and legal underpinnings for the care demonstrated in the second vignette were not available or well developed as recently as the 1990s, and in many hospitals, not even in the last decade. What has changed for surgeons in the interim is their growing capacity to respond to the complexity and potential of patients' experience of serious illness rather than narrowing the scope of the patient encounter by conceptualizing it as management of stage IV disease. Using the operation as the ultimate metaphor for surgeons, the physical operation used to manage a terminal situation in 1985 has evolved into a more expanded concept of the operation, an interdisciplinary exercise that restores comfort, dignity, and hope. This evolution could not

| Table 1<br>Palliative care definitions | |
|---|---|
| Palliative care | Medical care provided by an interdisciplinary team, including the professions of medicine, nursing, social work, chaplaincy, counseling, nursing assistant, and other health care professions, focused on the relief of suffering and support for the best possible quality of life for patients facing serious life-threatening illness and their families. It aims to identify and address the physical, psychological, spiritual, and practical burdens of illness.[45] |
| Palliative medicine | Palliative medicine is the study and management of patients with active, progressive, and far-advanced disease, for which the prognosis is limited and the focus of care is the quality of life.[46] |
| Surgical palliative care | *Surgical* palliative care is the treatment of suffering and the promotion of quality of life for patients who are seriously or terminally ill under surgical care.[1] |
| Palliative surgery | A surgical procedure used with the primary intention of improving quality of life or relieving symptoms caused by advanced disease. Its effectiveness is judged by the presence and durability of patient-acknowledged symptom resolution. |
| Hospice | *Hospice* is variably used to describe a (1) philosophy of care, (2) a place of care, or (3) an insurance benefit, such as the Medicare Hospice Benefit. Hospice describes supportive care for patients and their families during the patients' final phase of life-limiting illness. The traditional goal of hospice care is to enable patients to be comfortable and free of pain, so that they live each day as contentedly as possible. |

have occurred, however, without a concurrent shift in the public and the courts' perception of death.

## PALLIATIVE MEDICINE: ITS RECOGNITION AND LEGITIMIZATION IN MEDICAL PRACTICE

Palliative medicine was first recognized as a medical specialty in the United Kingdom where it evolved from the modern hospice movement that also began there during the 1960s and 1970s. It was recognized in Great Britain as a medical subspecialty as early as 1987. Balfour Mount, a urologic oncologist, established the world's first acute care hospital in-patient palliative care service at the Royal Victoria Hospital in Montreal in 1974. His prescient work anticipated the need for these services in an acute care (and surgical) environment that is only now being validated by outcomes studies. He coined the term, *palliative care*.[2] About that time, the first hospice program was established in the United States and the hospice movement was well established here before the field organized and differentiated itself sufficiently to evolve into a medical subspecialty.

The organizational beginnings of the specialty of hospice and palliative medicine in the United States occurred in 1988 when 250 physicians formed the Academy of Hospice Physicians. By the end of 1996, the organization had grown, changed its name to the American Academy of Hospice and Palliative Medicine (AAHPM), and sponsored the American Board of Hospice and Palliative Medicine (ABHPM). The

ABHPM independently gave its first certifying examination in November 1996. As of 2006, The American Board of Medical Specialties (ABMS) and its affiliated sponsoring boards have superseded the certification process previously sponsored by ABHPM.

In 2006, the AAHPM and the American Board of Hospice and Palliative Medicine jointly succeeded in achieving recognition of the subspecialty of hospice and palliative medicine within the ABMS and the Accreditation Council for Graduate Medical Education (ACGME). Ten ABMS boards, including the American Board of Surgery and the American Board of Anesthesiology, were subsequently authorized to confer ABMS certification for Hospice and Palliative Medicine. ABMS reported a total of 1271 physicians who successfully received subspecialty certification in hospice and palliative medicine from one of the 10 cosponsoring boards following the first examination in 2008.[3]

Currently, there are 26 surgeons and 58 anesthesiologists certified. Critical care and pain management, both very relevant to palliative care, are other subspecialty certifications available to American Board of Anesthesiology diplomates. Following the recognition of hospice and palliative medicine by ABMS and ACGME, The Center for Medicare and Medicaid Services followed suit in 2008. During the past several years, the number of fellowships in palliative medicine has increased (as of January 2010) to a total of 74 active programs offering 181 fellowship positions, including 27 research slots. ACGME has accredited 73 of these programs. After October 2012, only those who have completed an ACGME-accredited fellowship in palliative medicine will be able to sit for the ABMS certification examination. The small number of participants emerging from palliative medicine fellowships who could be certified and those currently certified will not be adequate to respond to the needs of the nation's increasing numbers of hospice and palliative care programs. The looming certified palliative specialist shortfall should prompt practicing physicians and surgeons who are not certified in palliative medicine to familiarize themselves with the basic principles and practices of palliative care as they apply to their respective disciplines. Because the number of surgeons and anesthesiologists who will pursue fellowships in hospice and palliative medicine will be small, surgeons will have to rely on nonsurgeon palliative medicine specialists for guidance in research design, quality improvement initiatives, and promotion of palliative care.

Other developments critical for the alignment of palliative care with mainstream medicine and positioning it for further introduction into the health care continuum has been the issuance of guidelines and preferred practices. In 2001, with foundation funding, The National Consensus Project for Quality Palliative Care initiative was launched with members representing the leading 5 hospice and palliative care organizations in the United States. Consensus guidelines were subsequently issued in 2004.[4] Using these guidelines as a foundation (**Box 1**), The National Quality Forum established its *National Framework and Preferred Practices for Palliative and Hospice Care.*[5]

The palliative care movement has been shaped and accelerated by changing demographics, failures of the current health care system, the strengthening of individual's autonomy in end-of-life matters in judicial opinion during the past 3 decades, and the favorable popular impact of the hospice movement. In addition, considerable investment by private philanthropic organizations, including the Robert Wood Johnson Foundation[6] and The Open Society Institute[7] founded by George Soros, provided the support necessary to develop the infrastructure and maintain the momentum of the field following the earlier success of hospice whose launching was also greatly benefited by private philanthropic funding before the passage of the Medicare Hospice Benefit in 1983. The success in leveraging millions of dollars of federal

---

**Box 1**
**National Quality Forum's 8 domains of quality palliative and hospice care**

1. Structures and processes of care
2. Physical aspects of care
3. Psychological and psychiatric aspects of care
4. Social aspects of care
5. Spiritual, religious, and existential aspects of care
6. Cultural aspects of care
7. Care of patients who are imminently dying
8. Ethical and legal aspects of care

*From* National Quality Forum. A national framework and preferred practices for palliative and hospice care quality. A consensus report. Washington, DC: National Quality Forum; 2006. Available at: http://www.qualityforum.org/Publications/2006/12/A_National_Framework_and_Preferred_Practices_for_Palliative_and_Hospice_Care_Quality.aspx. Accessed January 14, 2011; with permission.

---

support by the private sector for the dying stands out as an instructive and encouraging example for future initiatives related to revision of the health care system. Formerly rapidly fatal diseases, such as cancer, cardiovascular disease, and HIV, have become chronic, life-limiting illnesses. This development has contributed to the expansion of the elderly population that has contributed to the dramatically increasing and unsustainable per capita expenditures[8] for costly new technologies and drugs. An unforeseen consequence of technological success has been the fragmentation of medical care from the subspecialization that has accompanied these advances. This fragmentation is undermining primary care that has historically been the specialty of knowing the individual in their medical and social context. The erosion of primary care has too often left no effective physician advocate for patients in situations where vision and guidance far beyond the repertoire of surgery and medications are needed. Finally, there has been increased recognition of family caregivers and their unmet practical, social, and psychological needs.[9] Because of its patient/family focus; its emphasis on quality of life; and its recognition of the importance of social, psychological, and spiritual needs, palliative care appears suited to respond to many of these needs and to correct some of the failings of the current health care system.

Given these developments, palliative care programs have not surprisingly proliferated in the United States during the past decade. As of 2008, 53% of hospitals with more than 50 beds in the United States had a palliative care program.[10] Most of these are in-hospital programs, although nursing homes, outpatient treatment centers, and Veterans Affairs hospitals are offering these services. Two initiatives, the Center to Advance Palliative Care[11] and the Veterans Affairs Hospice and Palliative Care Initiative,[12] have greatly facilitated the introduction of palliative care into the in-hospital setting. As the concept has expanded across the spectrum of health care settings, it has also penetrated more than a dozen medical subspecialties in varying degrees whether through sponsorship of the American Board of Internal Medicine subspecialty certification in hospice and palliative medicine or attention to palliative care in position papers, specialty meetings, and journals.

One of the most notable trends, particularly relevant to surgeons and anesthesiologists, has been the acceptance of palliative care in the critical care setting (see article by Christine C. Toevs elsewhere in this issue for further exploration of this topic). This acceptance might have been inconceivable to many a decade ago, although certainly not surprising given the similarity of illness severity of patients served in the ICU and patients considered suitable for palliative care elsewhere. Palliative care and critical care have 4 fundamental similarities: (1) Both have a strong tradition of team-based care. (2) Both identify patients and families as a unit, which has been a longstanding precept of palliative care for philosophic reasons related to social and psychologic support of patients, while the patient/family is establishing itself as a treatment unit in critical care medicine because of the practical and legal necessity to turn to surrogates for direction and future care planning. Wall and colleagues[13] noted that family satisfaction in the ICU setting was higher for patients that died in the ICU than for families of survivors. They speculate that the increased attention by staff to families of non-survivors was the reason. (3) Both palliative care and critical care recognize that symptom control is mandatory for improvement of function even if only for the function of hope. (4) Both recognize and emphasize the role of communication. Good communication skills, a prerequisite for all palliative care, have recently received closer attention in critical care.[14] There is a high incidence (~30%) of posttraumatic stress disorder (PTSD) among families of ICU survivors, and evidence that the risk of PTSD can be ameliorated by communication with family before patients die or leave the ICU alive.[15] Two models of palliative care have been proposed for the ICU setting: the consultative model uses palliative care consultants to work with ICU staff to guide patients/families identified as not likely to survive the hospitalization and the integrative model seeks to incorporate palliative care principles and interventions in the daily practice of the intensive care unit team for all patients and families facing critical illness.[16]

For surgeons, burn care is the most obvious model for what critical palliative care should look like. It is an outstanding model for palliative care because the care of patients is not based on prognosis but their need for comfort while attempting to preserve or improve function. There is arguably no experience for patients who are critically ill that compares with a major burn for registering extremely high levels of distress in all dimensions of perception (physical, psychological, socioeconomic, and spiritual). Burns are truly a transformative experience for all involved for that reason and for some an end-of-life article. Until recently, burn care was the only surgical care where narcotics were routinely liberally and appropriately employed if for no other reason to make patients manageable and functional as they would be for patients receiving palliative care. This principle was established early on in the hospice movement: the relief of pain is a major prerequisite to the restoration of hope.

Over the past decade, increasing evidence has documented the social, psychological, economic, and even survival benefits for patients in the hospital and outpatient setting resulting from palliative care consultation and interventions. Palliative care has been shown to be patient-centered, beneficial, safe and not associated with earlier death, and more efficient in the use of health care resources and cost. Hospice care received substantially higher satisfaction ratings by families of decedents when compared with standard home health care, hospital care, and nursing home care.[9] Given this finding, it is not surprising that several studies have shown that palliative care improves pain and nonpain symptom control and family satisfaction with care in the public and Veterans' hospital settings.[17–20]

For years, palliative care professionals have suspected that palliative care improves survival in some patient populations. Several reasons could be invoked: avoidance of toxic nonbeneficial treatments, improved compliance with disease-directed treatments, and physiologic benefits resulting from effective symptom control (ie, relief of angina or dyspnea in patients with cardiomyopathy). In a 2007 study, the mean survival was 29 days longer for hospice patients than for nonhospice patients.[21] A recent study by Temel and colleagues[22] demonstrated early palliative care for patients with metastatic non-small–cell lung cancer is not only associated with significantly better quality of life, mood, and less aggressive treatment at end of life but also *increased survival*. Increased survival has been identified by Easson[23] as a potential outcome measure for palliative surgical procedures that had previously been recommended only for symptom control.

A significant factor in the rapid proliferation of hospital-based palliative care programs has no doubt been the cost avoidance realized by the reduction in hospital and ICU stays and costly invasive procedures resulting from effective palliative care team intervention. Not only has palliative care reduced hospital costs,[24] reduced days in the ICU and hospital,[25] it has also not been associated with increased mortality or morbidity. In some cases, the avoidance of invasive procedures that would have been performed on debilitated patients has probably increased their survival as well. The 30-day postoperative mortality and morbidity of patients with advanced cancer is considerable.[26] Despite these benefits, palliative care has not been timely[27] in the hospital setting.

Charles Von Gunten, currently Editor-in-Chief of *Palliative Medicine* and Chairman, Test Committee, Hospice and Palliative Medicine, American Board of Medical Specialties, and previous holder of many leadership positions in palliative care organizations, summarizes the change in palliative care over the past decade:

"To me, the most significant change is the move from palliative care as an 'option' or a 'choice' to proven gold standard of care that should be offered to all patients. We should be giving up any 'choice' language. It should all be focused now on 'how'." (Charles Von Gunten, MD, personal communication, September 9, 2010).

For an extensive and scholarly review of the growth and current status of palliative care in the United States, the reader is referred to Meier D. The development, status, and future of palliative care. In: Meier D, Isaacs SL, Hughes R, editors. Palliative care: transforming the care of serious illness. San Francisco: Jossey Bass; 2010. p. 1–464. Available at http://www.rwjf.org/files/research/4558.pdf.

See **Table 2** for a list of additional resources for surgeons interested in palliative care.

## SURGERY AND PALLIATIVE CARE: THE ROLE OF THE AMERICAN COLLEGE OF SURGEONS

Over the past 15 years, the American College of Surgeons has been the primary catalyst for the recognition of palliative care in the field of surgery, primarily through educational efforts. The college has also endorsed palliative care in a series of professional standards statements[28,29] and public policy recommendations.[30] Much credit is due to the personal interest of the highest level of the college's leadership and its Division of Education, the sustained efforts of Wendy Husser who initiated the surgical palliative care series for the *Journal of the American College of Surgeons*, and Linn Meyer who never missed an opportunity to advocate for palliative care through her administration of public relations outlets for the college. During the past 2 decades, the college's perspective on end-of-life matters has evolved from debating physician-assisted suicide (PAS) in the mid to late 1990s to recognizing and implementing clinical approaches to palliative care in the current decade. No matter what position was taken in the physician-assisted suicide debate, it did little to improve symptom relief and clinical guidance for thousands of patients and families with life-limiting illness.

| Table 2 |
| --- |
| **Palliative care education resources for surgeons** |

| | |
| --- | --- |
| Center to Advance Palliative Care<br>Available at: http://www.capc.org/ | The Center to Advance Palliative Care provides health care professionals with tools, training, and technical assistance necessary to start and sustain palliative care programs in hospitals and other health care settings |
| Education of Physicians about End-of-Life Care<br>Available at: http://www.eperc.mcw.edu/ | This site has been designed for use by medical school course/clerkship directors, residency, and continuing education program directors, medical faculty, community preceptors, or other professionals who are (or will be) involved in providing end-of-life instruction to health care professionals in training |
| Dunn G, Martensen R, Weissman D, editors<br>*Surgical palliative care: A resident's guide*<br>Chicago:<br>American College of Surgeons. Cuniff-Dixon Foundation; 2009<br>Available through<br>American College of Surgeons<br>633 N, St Clair Street<br>Chicago, IL 60,611–3211 | Guide introducing surgeons in training to the basic principles and practices of surgical palliative care |
| Hospice and Palliative Care Training for Physicians: UNIPAC, 3rd edition<br>American Academy of hospice and Palliative Medicine<br>Available at: http://www.aahpm.org/resources/default/training.html | 9 module self-study program for physicians, which introduces hospice and palliative care concepts and practices for a variety of patient groups (cancer, chronic obstructive pulmonary disease, dementia, HIV/AIDS, pediatrics |
| Walsh D, Caraceni AT, Fainsinger R, et al, editors<br>*Palliative Medicine*. Philadelphia: Saunders-Elsevier; 2009 | Hardbound and online textbook of palliative medicine with contributions from many pioneers of the specialty |

In the late 1990s, most surgeons would have equated end-of-life care with hospice, PAS, or medical ethics. Since then, a broader understanding of the relevance of quality-of-life outcomes to day-to-day decision making and treatments for patients who are seriously ill has emerged. This understanding is reflected in 2 position statements of the college in 1998 and 2005. The first statement refers specifically to end of life and hospice, reinforcing the impression that palliative care is something that happens in the last stages of life. The subsequent statement is framed in language that adapts palliative principles to a much more broad population for whom death is not imminent or certain but for whom distress is likely, such as those in a critical care setting or with a new diagnosis of cancer. Currently, the college is focusing on the education of surgeons and surgeons in training in the strategy and tactics of palliative care, communication, and symptom management (**Box 2**),[31] while not abandoning its long-standing attention to medical ethics.[32] A recent important contribution of the college's Commission on Cancer has been the addition of a new Cancer Program Standard for 2012 that states, "Palliative care services are available to patients on-site or by referral."[33]

---

**Box 2**
**List of teaching modules in surgical palliative care: a resident's guide**

- Personal awareness, self-care, and the surgeon-patient relationship
- Pain
- Dyspnea
- Delirium
- Depression
- Nausea
- Constipation
- Malignant bowel obstruction
- Cachexia, anorexia, asthenia, fatigue (wasting syndromes)
- Artificial nutrition and hydration
- Palliative surgery: definition, principles, outcomes assessment
- Pediatric palliative care
- Cross-cultural encounters
- Delivering bad news
- Goals of care/conducting a family conference
- The do not resuscitate discussion
- Palliative and hospice care referrals
- Care during the final days of life
- Discussing spiritual issues: maintaining hope

*From* Dunn G, Martensen R, Weissman D, editors. Surgical palliative care: a resident's guide. Chicago: American College of Surgeons. Cuniff-Dixon Foundation; 2009; with permission.

---

To summarize the college's contribution to the evolution of surgical palliative care over the past 2 decades, it started with its search for an effective strategy for the care of patients at the end of life following the establishment of the legal pathway to freedom from futile or undesired treatments as laid out in the landmark cases of Quinlan[34] (ruling allowed withdrawal of ventilator support from patient in permanent vegetative state), Cruzan[35] (ruling affirmed that patients who could not make decisions still retained a right to refuse medical treatment), and its acknowledgment of end-of-life issues within the limited scope of the physician-assisted suicide debate. From the previous highly intellectualized ethical discourse evolved a more practical concern about how surgeons should communicate with patients who are seriously ill, how they should manage their most troubling symptoms, and how they can contribute to the restoration of hope using their own and their patients' personal, socioeconomic, and spiritual assets. Growing public interest and awareness of end-of-life issues and its implications for future health policy advocacy has catalyzed this transition.

## PALLIATIVE CARE AND THE AMERICAN BOARD OF SURGERY

The American Board of Surgery was one of 10 boards of the American Board of Medical Specialties that sponsored the formation of the subspecialty of Hospice and Palliative Medicine in 2006. A small number of surgeons have been certified to date. Up until now 2 paths to certification have been open to surgeons seeking certification in hospice and palliative medicine: experiential and fellowship. The window for grandfathering is closing, as the required 2-year period of affiliation with a hospice or palliative care team has already started for those attempting to sit for the next (2012) examination. Following 2012, completion of an ACGME-credited palliative medicine fellowship program will be required to sit for the examination. The American Board of Anesthesiology has similar requirements. Apart from offering a certification in hospice and palliative medicine, the American Board of Surgery considers palliative care skills among the expected domains of competence for surgeons seeking board certification.[36]

## SURGICAL PALLIATIVE CARE ACROSS THE SPECTRUM OF SURGERY

Currently, the concept of surgical palliative care appears to be establishing itself in critical and trauma care mainly because of the similarities of palliative care and critical care as previously outlined. Access to palliative care in that setting is still quite limited and not improved by use of triggers to prompt palliative care referrals.[37] However, a recent presentation[38] at the American College of Surgeons' 96th Annual Clinical Congress demonstrated the compatibility of palliative care for transplantation patients in all stages of the transplantation continuum. In a recent study, trauma-burn surgeons and neurosurgeons reported being better equipped to manage multidimensional suffering of patients with sudden advanced illness when collaborating with a palliative care team.[39] Jacobs and colleagues[40] published a best-practice model for end-of-life support for trauma patients and their families. It stands as a model for the application of surgical palliative care in other venues beyond trauma care because it is a systems-based and interdisciplinary model. The American Trauma Society has published a valuable contribution to surgical palliative care in *The Second Trauma Program. The Art of Communicating with Families of Trauma Patients*.[41] The *second trauma* that the title refers to is the emotional trauma that happens to the family of the victim, the *first trauma* is the injury to the victim. The manual outlines communication and support techniques and strategies. It also addresses specific issues, such as family support after suicide, requests for organ donation, family presence during resuscitation, and suspected abuse.

The field of surgical oncology has seen a consensus and refinement of the definition of palliative surgery (see **Table 1**). The definition that has emerged is now in alignment with palliative as understood by the rest of the field of palliative care. Other contributions will include increased use of less invasive surgical techniques and better prognostication, especially for those patients for whom operative intervention is being considered. A nomogram has recently been developed to predict 30-day morbidity and mortality for patients with disseminated malignancy undergoing surgical intervention.[42] This type of innovation will be a valuable adjunct to the developing field of communication. The social, ethical, and statistical complexity of designing clinical trials for palliative surgical outcomes[43,44] will benefit from the extensive experience and work that has been done in nonsurgical palliative care research.

## SURGICAL PALLIATIVE CARE: WILL IT TRANSFORM SURGERY AND SURGEONS?

What will successful implementation of palliative care in the field of surgery look like? It will be successfully established when any surgical patient who is seriously ill and their family know to request palliative care; all surgeons have the willingness, knowledge, and skills to ensure their patients will receive palliative care; and the surgical venue will be prepared and equipped to provide palliative care. This success will require not only a change in the cognitive and technical repertoire of the surgeon but also a change of the surgical character that is willing to risk some degree of psychologic and spiritual reflection and introspection. In the past, surgeons have made similarly significant adjustments. The eighteenth century surgeon who relied on speed and callousness to accomplish life-saving amputations yielded to the more deliberate, cerebral, and gentler surgeon of the late nineteenth and twentieth century who performed reconstructions. It seems particularly appropriate in the current era of social networking and globalization to ask if the surgeon of the twenty-first century be noted for their ability to recognize the impact of their intervention beyond the merely physical aspects the patients' experience and its impact beyond the individual patient.

Palliative care is not care for the dying, but care of people with serious or life-limiting illness, some of whom will die imminently. To limit the concept of palliative care to the dying only reinforces the current Western dichotomous view of life and death, which could be summarized as all or nothing or fight or flight. The richness of palliative care lies in its recognition of the possible where there is uncertainty. There is nothing uncertain about robust health or active dying. This philosophy is an extension of the hospice philosophy that has facilitated the transition from *death as failure* to *dying as opportunity*. For those who actually are at the end of their life, palliative care offers the opportunity to die in peace instead of pieces. For those not at the end of life, palliative care offers the same hope: to live in peace, not piecemeal. The specialties of surgery and anesthesiology have too many seriously ill people in its care and has too much to offer the seriously ill with all diagnoses to not assume a leadership role for the continued growth and development of palliative care. Recent developments in the field of surgery and the anticipated development of this idea in the field of anesthesiology give reason for optimism that this will occur.

## REFERENCES

1. Dunn G. Surgical palliative care. In: Cameron J, editor. Current surgical therapy. 9th edition. Philadelphia: Mosby, Elsevier; 2008. p. 1179.
2. Clemens KE, Jaspers B, Klaschik E. The history of hospice. In: Walsh D, Caraceni AT, Fainsinger R, et al, editors. Palliative medicine. Philadelphia: Saunders-Elsevier; 2009. p. 20.
3. Available at: http://www.aahpm.org/certification/abms.html. Accessed September 12, 2010.
4. National Consensus Project for Quality Palliative Care. Clinical practice guidelines (2004). Available at: http://www.nationalconsensusproject.org/Guidelines_Download.asp. Accessed January 13, 2011.
5. National Quality Forum. A national framework and preferred practices for palliative and hospice care; December 2006. Available at: http://www.qualityforum.org/publications/reports/palliative.asp. Accessed January 13, 2011.
6. Bronner E. The foundation's end of life programs: changing the American way of death. To improve health and health care, vol. vi: the Robert Wood Johnson Foundation anthology. San Francisco (CA): Jossey-Bass; 2003.
7. McGlinchey L, editor. Transforming the culture of dying: the project on death in America. New York: Open Society Institute; 2004. p. 1–72.
8. Poisal JA, Truffer C, Smith C, et al. Health spending projections through 2016: modest changes obscure part D's impacts. Health Aff 2007;26:W242–53.
9. Teno JM, Clarridge BR, Casey V, et al. Family perspectives on end-of-life care at the last place of care. JAMA 2004;291:88–93.

10. Center to Advance Palliative Care. National palliative care research center. America's care of serious illness: a state-by-state report card on access to palliative care in our nation's hospitals. Available at: http://www.capc.org/reportcard/state-by-state-report-card.pdf. Accessed, January 14, 2011.

11. Center to Advance Palliative Care. Palliative care NCP guidelines-center to advance palliative care. Available at: http://www.capc.org/ncp-guidelines/view?searchterm=clinical%20practice%20guidelines. Accessed January 14, 2011.

12. Office of Geriatrics and Extended Care. US department of veteran's affairs. hospice and palliative care. Available at: http://www1.va.gov/GERIATRICS/Hospice_Palliative_Care2.asp. Accessed January 14, 2011.

13. Wall RJ, Curtis JR, Cooke CR, et al. Family satisfaction in the ICU: differences between families of survivors and nonsurvivors. Chest 2007;132(5):1425–33.

14. Curtis JR, White DB. Practical guidance for evidence-based ICU family conferences. Chest 2008;134(4):835–43.

15. Azoulay E, Pochard F, Kentish-Barnes N, et al. Risk of post-traumatic stress symptoms in family members of intensive care unit patients. Am J Respir Crit Care Med 2005;171(9):987–94.

16. Nelson JE, Bassett R, Boss RD, et al. Models for structuring a clinical initiative to enhance palliative care in the intensive care unit: a report from the IPAL-ICU Project (improving palliative care in the ICU). Crit Care Med 2010;38(9):1765–72.

17. Higginson IJ, Finlay I, Goodwin DM, et al. Do hospital-based palliative teams improve care for patients or families at the end of life? J Pain Symptom Manage 2002;23:96–106.

18. Higginson IJ, Finlay IG, Goodwin DM, et al. Is there evidence that palliative care teams alter end-of-life experiences of patients and their caregivers? J Pain Symptom Manage 2003;25:150–68.

19. Finlay IG, Higginson IJ, Goodwin DM, et al. Palliative care in hospital, hospice, at home: results from a systematic review. Ann Oncol 2002;13(Suppl 4):257–64.

20. Casarett D, Pickard A, Bailey FA, et al. Do palliative care consultations improve patient outcomes? J Am Geriatr Soc 2008;56(4):593–9.

21. Connor SR, Pyenson B, Fitch K, et al. Comparing hospice and non-hospice patient survival among patients who die within a three year window. J Pain Symptom Manage 2007;33(3):238–46.

22. Temel JS, Greer JA, Muzikansky A, et al. Early palliative care for patients with metastatic non-small-cell lung cancer. N Engl J Med 2010;363(8):733–42.

23. Cady B, Barker F, Easson A. Part 3: surgical palliation of advanced illness: what's new, what's helpful. J Am Coll Surg 2005;200(3):457–66.

24. Penrod JD, Deb P, Dellenbaugh C, et al. Hospital-based palliative care consultation: effects on hospital cost. J Palliat Med 2010;13(8):973–9.

25. Ciemins EL, Blum L, Nunley M, et al. The economic and clinical impact of an inpatient palliative care consultation service. J Palliat Med 2007;10:1347–55.

26. Cady B, Miner T, Morgentaler A. Part 2: surgical palliation of advanced illness: what's new, what's helpful. J Am Coll Surg 2005;200(2):281–90.

27. Penrod JD, Deb P, Luhrs C, et al. Cost and utilization outcomes of patients receiving hospital-based palliative care consultation. J Palliat Med 2006;9(4):855–60 [erratum in: J Palliat Med 2006;9(6):1509].

28. American College of Surgeons Committee on Ethics. Statement of principles guiding care at the end of life. Bull Am Coll Surg 1998;83(4):46.

29. American College of Surgeons Committee on Ethics and Surgical Palliative Care Task Force. Statement of principles of palliative care. Bull Am Coll Surg 2005; 90(8):34–45.

30. American College of Surgeons. Statement on health care reform. Bull Am Coll Surg 2008;93:1–5.
31. Dunn G, Martensen R, Weissman D, editors. Surgical palliative care: a resident's guide. American college of surgeons. Chicago: Cuniff-Dixon Foundation; 2009. p. 107–32.
32. McGrath MH, Risucci DA, Schwab A, editors. Ethical issues in clinical surgery. Chicago: American College of Surgeons; 2007. p. 1–149.
33. Commission on Cancer. Cancer Program Standards 2012. American College of Surgeons. Chicago, in press.
34. In Re Quinlan, 355 A.2d 647 (N.J. 1976).
35. Cruzan v Missouri Department of Health, 497 U.S. 261 (1990).
36. Available at: http://home.absurgery.org/xfer/BookletofInfo-Surgery.pdf. Accessed January 13, 2011.
37. Bradley C, Weaver J, Brasel K. Addressing access to palliative care services in the surgical intensive care unit. Surgery 2010;147(6):871–7.
38. Aloia TA. Syndrome of imminent demise. Panel session 219: common problems and quality outcomes: surgical care for the terminal patient. American College of Surgeons 96th Annual Clinical Congress. Washington, DC, October 5, 2010.
39. Tilden LB, Williams BR, Tucker RO, et al. Surgeons' attitudes and practices in the utilization of palliative and supportive care services for patients with a sudden advanced illness. Palliat Med 2009;12(11):1037–42.
40. Jacobs BB, Jacobs LM, Burns K. Trauma end of life optimum support. A best practice model for trauma professionals. Woodbury (CT): CineMed Publishing, Inc; 2010. p. 1–127.
41. Cronin M, Kelly P, Lipton, et al. The 2nd trauma program. The art of communicating with families of trauma patients. Upper Marlboro (MD): American Trauma Society; 2006. p. 1–50.
42. Tseng WH, Yang XY, Wang H, et al. Nomogram to predict risk of 30-day morbidity and mortality for patients with disseminated malignancy undergoing surgical intervention. Presented at the American Society of Clinical Oncology Annual Meeting. Chicago, June 4–8, 2010.
43. Mularski RA, Rosenfeld K, Coons SJ, et al. Measuring outcomes in randomized prospective trials in palliative care. J Pain Symptom Manage 2007;34(Suppl 1):S7–19.
44. Krouse RS, Easson AM, Angelos P. Ethical considerations and barriers to research in surgical palliative care. J Am Coll Surg 2003;196(3):469–74.
45. National Consensus Project. Clinical practice guidelines for quality palliative care. 2009. Available at: http://www.nationalconsensusproject.org. Accessed September 12, 2010.
46. Doyle D, Hanks G, Cherny N. Introduction. In: Doyle D, Hanks G, Cherny N, et al, editors. Oxford textbook of palliative medicine. 3rd edition. Oxford (UK): Oxford University Press; 2004. p. 1.

# Palliative Medicine in the Surgical Intensive Care Unit and Trauma

Christine C. Toevs, MD, FACS, FCCM

## KEYWORDS

- Palliative care • Trauma • Surgical intensive care unit
- End of life • Family support • Communication

Palliative Medicine is a new discipline that focuses on all aspects of a person in relation to medicine: physical, spiritual, and emotional. The purpose of palliative medicine is to prevent and relieve suffering and to help patients and their families set informed goals of care and treatment. Palliative medicine can be provided along with life-prolonging treatment or as the main focus of treatment.

The intensive care unit (ICU) plays a prominent role in medical care in the United States today. National data suggest 30% to 40% of all patients admitted to the ICU will die while in the ICU or before hospital discharge, and 22% of all deaths in the United States now occur in or after admission to an ICU. Palliative medicine has an increasing role and presence in the ICU. The purpose of this article is to discuss the growing and essential role of palliative medicine to comprehensive patient-centered care in the surgical intensive care unit (SICU) and trauma.

## LONG-TERM OUTCOMES IN SICU AND TRAUMA

In the past several years, studies have begun to address the long-term outcomes of patients following ICU admission. Wunsch and colleagues[1] looked at 35,308 Medicare ICU subjects who survived to hospital discharge. They noted that ICU survivors had higher 3-year mortality (39.5%) than hospital controls (34.5%). ICU subjects who had received mechanical ventilation had substantially increased mortality at 3 years (57.6%). Most of the ventilated subjects died in the first 6 months after ICU admission (30.1% vs 9.6% for hospital controls). They concluded that an increase in mortality was present for 3 years after ICU admission.

In Australia, Williams and associates looked at all adult subjects admitted to the ICU who survived to hospital discharge.[2] They noted the risk of death for these

---

A version of this article was published in the 91.2 issue of *Surgical Clinics of North America*.
The author has nothing to disclose.
Allegheny General Hospital, 320 East North Avenue, Pittsburgh, PA 15212, USA
*E-mail address:* ctoevs@aol.com

Anesthesiology Clin 30 (2012) 29–35
doi:10.1016/j.anclin.2011.11.002
1932-2275/12/$ – see front matter © 2012 Elsevier Inc. All rights reserved.

**anesthesiology.theclinics.com**

subjects was higher than the general public for 15 years after ICU admission. They concluded that an episode of critical illness, or its treatment, may shorten life expectancy.

In Germany, Schneider and colleagues[3] looked specifically at long-term survival after surgical critical illness. They followed 1462 subjects with an ICU stay of greater than 4 days, until the end of the second year after ICU admission. Of the 1055 subjects (72.0%) discharged from the ICU, 808 (55.3%) survived 6 months, and at 2 years 648 (44.3%) subjects were alive. They concluded that survivors of surgical critical illness suffer from a post-ICU syndrome. They stated, "specific sequelae of critical illness may create a defined constellation of signs and symptoms that are both directly attributable to the episode of preceding critical illness and responsible for morbidity and mortality beyond the underlying disease."[3]

Dialysis is a frequent intervention started in the intensive care unit setting. As the population grows older, so does the age of patients in the ICU; more patients are being admitted from nursing home settings. Tamura and colleagues[4] studied hospitalized subjects in nursing homes with end-stage renal disease and the initiation of dialysis. At 12 months after initiation of dialysis, 58% of these subjects had died and predialysis functional status was maintained in only 13%. These were subjects with single-organ failure at the start of dialysis. Often ICU patients have multiple-organ failure, of which renal failure is just one component, supporting the poor outcomes of these patients after the initiation of dialysis.

In Norway, Halverson[5] recommends that discussions about starting dialysis in the elderly population should involve the health care team and patients. He suggests a transparent discussion, involving the difficult decisions of withdrawing and withholding dialysis, should occur before initiation of dialysis. He also states that medicine tends to focus on the technical aspects of dialysis and neglects the overall needs of patients. Furthermore, consent involves only the technical components of the procedure and not in the context of overall outcomes of patients. This trend of technical procedural-based consent, rather than contextual informed consent is more common in elderly patients because the complexities of their needs are greater than younger patients.

Increasingly, hospitals and ICUs have been using long-term acute care hospitals (LTACs) to facilitate recovery from a critical illness. However, the outcomes of these patients being transferred to LTACs are rarely communicated to the patients and families. The 1-year survival of Medicare beneficiaries transferred to an LTAC is 52%.[6] In their study, Kahn and associates commented that we need strategies "to improve both prognosis and communication about prognosis to ensure decision makers do not have unreasonable expectations surrounding long-term acute care."[6]

Regarding trauma patients specifically, in New Jersey, Livingston and associates[7] evaluated the long-term outcomes of trauma subjects admitted to the SICU. They contacted 100 subjects who experienced trauma with ICU stays greater than 10 days. A total of 81 subjects were men with a mean age of 42 years. Traumatic brain injury was present in 50 subjects. The mean follow-up was 3.3 years from discharge. They noted that only 49% of subjects were back to work or school following injury. They noted ICU survivors greater than 3 years after severe injury have significant impairments, including inability to return to work. They stated, "The goal of reintegrating patients back into society is not being met." They concluded that although survival is an important outcome after injury, it is not a sufficient outcome to measure success of a trauma center.

## DO NOT RESUSCITATE AND THE ICU

Physicians tend not to discuss do-not-resuscitate (DNR) orders with their patients. In New York, Sulmasy[8] surveyed doctors about their attitudes and confidence regarding DNR discussions. They noted physician confidence regarding DNR discussion is low compared with other medical discussions, such as procedural consent. They concluded that this lack of confidence in physicians having these discussions may contribute to the low occurrence rate of these conversations. Their study again supports the data that physicians' conversations with families tend to focus on technical aspects of treatment as opposed to long-term outcomes and contextual conversations based on goals of care.

Cardiopulmonary resuscitation (CPR) in an ICU setting is rarely effective in providing long-term survival and survival to hospital discharge. Myrianthefs and colleagues[9] looked at subjects (111 total) who underwent CPR in an adult ICU. The 24-hour survival of subjects was 9.2%. The survival to discharge was 0. They recommended that DNR orders should be applied more frequently in the ICU.

Surgical services tend to discuss DNR less frequently than medical services. Morrell and colleagues[10] in Indiana compared the use of DNR orders in medical subjects versus surgical subjects at time of hospital death. They noted DNR orders were more frequent on medical subjects (77.3%) than surgical subjects (64.2%). This study showed these orders were made earlier in the hospital stay for medical subjects (9.8 days before death) rather than for surgical subjects (5.1 days before death). They concluded that DNR orders are typically written late in the patients' hospital course on both medical and surgical services. They also noted several previous studies, in which DNR orders in patients who died were written within 3 days of the subjects' deaths. They concluded that physicians still are reluctant to have these emotional and time-intensive conversations with patients and their families, thus contributing to the palliative medicine initiative.

## END-OF-LIFE CARE IN SICU AND TRAUMA

In 2008, the American Academy of Critical Care Medicine published a consensus statement on their recommendations for end-of-life (EOL) care in the ICU.[11] They recommended intensivists should be competent in all aspects of end-of-life care, including the "practical and ethical aspects of withdrawing different modalities of life-sustaining treatment and the use of sedatives, analgesics and nonpharmacologic approaches to easing the suffering of the dying process." Evidence supports "improved communication with the family has been shown to improve patient care and family outcomes."[11]

Communication in the ICU around EOL issues remains problematic. Lautrette and colleagues[12] reviewed the literature regarding end-of-life family conferences. They noted multiple studies demonstrating proactive interventions are needed to improve communication at the end of life. They note families want better communication because improved communication improves the care of patients. They state these studies show families need more support than informal family conferences. Families require assistance in understanding the information provided, support during the decision-making process, and assistance with alleviating their guilt. Families also require assistance with achieving consensus among family members even when a health care proxy has been designated. These family meetings are time intensive, supporting the role of teams dedicated to patient and family support.

Part of the problem may lie in the ICU model of open versus closed intensive care units. Cassell and colleagues[13] looked at the comparison of administrative models of ICUs and the interactions of medical personnel and families. They noted that when surgeons have primary responsibility for patients, the most important goal is "defeating death."[13] When intensivists have sole patient responsibility (closed ICU model) then quality of life and scarcity of resources are considered. Their conclusions state the administrative models of ICU care need to be evaluated. Physician behavior will not change until the ICU model of care is addressed regardless of education of EOL principles.

One suggestion to improve communication in the ICU is a simple checklist on ICU admission. Mularski[14] proposed a checklist that would identify surrogate decision makers and explore goals of care from a patient-family perspective. Application and quality could be measured by increased documentation of patient goals and preferences in the medical record. A checklist, however, does not ensure that difficult and emotional conversations occur and that information is appropriately relayed to patients and families. Often, a more structured team approach as provided by palliative care services is needed in this process.

## INTEGRATION OF A PALLIATIVE CARE TEAM

The medical intensive care unit (MICU) has already begun to investigate integrating the palliative medicine team into the ICU in certain situations. Campbell and Guzman,[15] at Wayne State University in Detroit, Michigan, compared ICU patients with end stage dementia who had a palliative medicine consult with those patients who did not have a palliative medicine consult. They noted a decreased hospital and MICU length of stay in subjects proactively identified with dementia and provided consultation from palliative medicine. They also noted that a "proactive palliative intervention decreased the time between identification of poor prognosis and the establishment of DNR goals, decreased time terminal demented subjects remained in the ICU, and reduced the use of nonbeneficial resources."[15] They stated that these interventions resulted in reduced burden and cost of care to the subjects and their families with increasing comfort and psycho-emotional support. There was no difference in the mortality or discharge to nursing home versus home in the 2 groups. In their study, palliative medicine consultation resulted in decreased length of stay and shorter time to defining goals of care without increasing mortality.

A similar study was done in the MICU in Rochester, New York. Norton and her team identified 191 subjects who, on admission to the MICU, had a high risk of dying.[16] Two-thirds of these subjects had palliative care consultation. Their data showed that subjects in the palliative care consultation group had a significantly shorter length of stay in the MICU, without a difference in total length of stay in the hospital. There were no differences in mortality rates or discharge disposition between the groups. They concluded that there is a growing body of literature suggesting that "proactive interventions focused on enhancing communication regarding patients' goals of care and benefits verses burdens of treatment are associated with shortened lengths of stay"[16] in the ICU.

In New York, O'Mahony and colleagues[17] published a descriptive study of the logistics of integration of the palliative care team into the ICUs at their hospitals. The advance practice nurse on the palliative care team went to the ICU daily to communicate with the ICU team. The palliative care team was consulted on one-third of the subjects that ultimately died within the ICU. They noted that subjects and families who had a consult had increased communication, education on the death process, improvements in pain and symptom management, increase in formalization of advance directives, and decrease in laboratory and radiology tests. Survival times were identical between the subjects that had palliative care involvement verses those who did not.

The SICU in Milwaukee tried to establish the use of triggers for increasing access to palliative care. Bradley and colleagues[18] identified subjects who would benefit from palliative care consultation as those who had a family request, futility considered or declared by medical team, family disagreement lasting more than 7 days, death expected during the same SICU stay, SICU stay greater than 1 month, diagnosis with median survival less than 6 months, greater than 3 SICU admissions during same hospitalization, Glasgow Coma Scale of less than 8 for more than 1 week in subjects aged younger than 75 years, and multiorgan failure in greater than 3 systems. Despite these triggers and identification of these subjects, the consult was at the discretion of the primary service or the SICU service in this ICU model. They noted that the use of triggers successfully identifies the subjects who were at a high risk of poor outcome (>50% mortality). However, the use of palliative care consults did not increase during the time period the triggers were implemented because the consult was optional and not mandatory. They suggested the daily use of a "palliative care bundle"[18] by the SICU team that addresses symptom control, goal setting and prognostication, psychosocial and spiritual support, advance care planning, and patient and family support, may improve outcomes for the patients in the SICU. They also suggested this bundle may work best in a closed ICU model.

Even with trauma patients in the ICU, a structured approach to palliative intervention was found to be beneficial. In New Jersey, Mosenthal and associates[19] instituted a palliative program implemented by the trauma surgeons and ICU nursing. This program included, on admission to the SICU, family bereavement support and assessment of prognosis and patient preferences. Secondly, they implemented interdisciplinary family meetings within 72 hours of admission. They noted the implementation of a palliative program did not change mortality, DNR, or withdraw of life-sustaining therapy rates, but both DNR and withdraw were implemented earlier in the hospital course. Of the patients who died, the ICU length of stay was decreased, and the time from DNR order to death was increased. They concluded that structured communication between physicians and families resulted in earlier consensus around goals of care for dying trauma patients. Integrating an early structured palliative program resulted in improved communication with families and improvement of EOL care.

The University of Rochester Medical Center launched an initiative to provide early consultation with palliative care for patients with severe traumatic brain injury.[20] They noted earlier and more thorough discussions with families about prognosis, patients' values, and outcomes occurred after routine palliative care consultation. They noted a small but significant decrease in tracheostomies performed in this patient population and an increase in withdraw of mechanical ventilation before tracheostomy. They noted that the integration of a palliative care team resulted in increased conversations with families "about the delicate, complex and emotionally demanding decisions required to achieve fully informed choice in life-changing, unfamiliar and often terrifying situations." They also noted medicine needs to move toward "more systematic conversations about the potential for invasive medical treatments both to do good and to harm patients toward the end of life."[20]

Recommendations for improving the quality of EOL care have been proposed by Nelson.[21] She stated the goals of integrating palliative care in the ICU are to optimize comfort and function for patients at all stages of serious and life-threatening disease. Integrating palliative care on admission to the ICU provided emotional and practical support for families, beginning at diagnosis of critical illness, regardless of prognosis.

In this model, palliative care is part of comprehensive critical care, not as an optional alternative, and is simultaneous with critical care rather than sequential. Patients can continue treatments with the goal of restoring health, and there is not an expectation that critical illness will result in death. Rather than trying to change the attitudes in society and medicine toward death, the emphasis is on transforming the experience of dying in the ICU.

## SUMMARY

As the population ages, the age of patients within the ICU also increases. In many of these clinical situations of trauma and postoperative surgical care, we do not adequately address the goals of care with patients and their families. An early integrated approach of palliative medicine in the SICU and trauma would offer patients and families improved communication of goals of care and support. Identification of evidence-based triggers for palliative medicine consults would facilitate this process (dialysis, tracheostomy in traumatic brain injury, dementia, ventilator >7 days, and so forth). Palliative medicine in the ICU offers the opportunity to decrease length of stay and decrease nonbeneficial resource use without increasing mortality. Taking care of our patients and their families and addressing all of their needs and goals, not just the physical, should be the role of every intensivist and surgeon.

## ACKNOWLEDGMENTS

The author sincerely thanks Ellen Harvey, MN, RN, CCRN, CNS, for her editorial assistance.

## REFERENCES

1. Wunsch H, Guerra C, Barnato A, et al. Three-year outcomes for Medicare beneficiaries who survive intensive care. JAMA 2010;303:849–56.
2. Williams T, Dobb G, Finn J, et al. Determinants of long-term survival after intensive care. Crit Care Med 2008;36:1523–30.
3. Schneider C, Fertmann J, Geiger S, et al. Long-term survival after surgical critical illness: the impact of prolonged preceding organ support therapy. Ann Surg 2010;251:1145–53.
4. Tamara M, Covinsky K, Chertow G, et al. Functional status of elderly adults before and after initiation of dialysis. N Engl J Med 2009;361:1539–47.
5. Halvorsen k, Slettebo A, Nortbedt P, et al. Priority dilemmas in dialysis: the impact of old age. J Med Ethics 2008;34:585–9.
6. Kahn J, Benson N, Appleby D, et al. Long-term acute care hospital utilization after critical illness. JAMA 2010;303:2253–9.
7. Livingston D, Tripp T, Biggs C, et al. A fate worse than death? Long-term outcome of trauma patients admitted to the surgical intensive care unit. J Trauma 2009;67: 341–9.
8. Sulmasy D, Sood J, Ury W. Physicians' confidence in discussion do not resuscitate orders with patients and surrogates. J Med Ethics 2008;34:96–101.
9. Myrianthefs P, Kalafati M, Lemonidou C, et al. Efficacy of CPR in a general adult ICU. Resuscitation 2003;57:43–8.
10. Morrell E, Brown B, Qi R, et al. The do-not-resuscitate order: associations with advance directives, physician specialty and documentation of discussion 15 years after the Patient Self-Determination Act. J Med Ethics 2008;34:642–7.

11. Truog R, Campbell M, Curtis J, et al. Recommendation for end-of-life care in the intensive care unit: a consensus statement by the American Academy of Critical Care Medicine. Crit Care Med 2008;36:953–63.
12. Lautrette A, Ciroldi M, Ksibi H, et al. End-of-life family conferences: rooted in the evidence. Crit Care Med 2006;34(Suppl):S364–72.
13. Cassell J, Buckman T, Streat S, et al. Surgeons, intensivists, and the covenant of care: administrative models and values affecting care at the end of life. Crit Care Med 2003;31:1263–70.
14. Mularski R. Defining and measuring quality palliative and end-of-life care in the intensive care unit. Crit Care Med 2006;34(Suppl):S309–16.
15. Campbell M, Guzman J. A proactive approach to improve end-of-life care in a medical intensive care unit for patients with terminal dementia. Crit Care Med 2004;32:1839–43.
16. Norton S, Hogan L, Holloway R, et al. Proactive palliative care in the medical intensive care unit: effects on length of stay for selected high-risk patients. Crit Care Med 2007;35:1530–5.
17. O'Mahony S, McHenry J, Blank A, et al. Preliminary report of the integration of a palliative care team into an intensive care unit. Palliat Med 2010;24:154–65.
18. Bradley C, Weaver J, Brasel K. Addressing access to palliative care services in the surgical intensive care unit. Surgery 2010;147:871–7.
19. Mosenthal A, Murphy P, Barker L, et al. Changing the culture around end-of-life care in the trauma intensive care unit. J Trauma 2008;64:1587–93.
20. Holloway R, Quill T. Treatment decisions after brain injury – tensions among quality, preference and cost. N Engl J Med 2010;362:1757–9.
21. Nelson J. Identifying and overcoming the barriers to high-quality palliative care in the intensive care unit. Crit Care Med 2006;34(Suppl):S324–31.

# Care of the Family in the Surgical Intensive Care Unit

Leslie Steele Tyrie, MD[a], Anne Charlotte Mosenthal, MD[b],*

**KEYWORDS**

- Surgical intensive care unit • Palliative care • Family support
- Surrogate decision maker • Communication

One of the subtle but important shifts in surgical palliative care from usual surgical care is the treatment of the family and patient as the unit of care. Nowhere is this more apparent than in the surgical intensive care unit (SICU), where the stress of having a critically ill loved one creates significant bereavement and emotional needs for family members. Multiple studies have now demonstrated that families of patients in the ICU are themselves in crisis, with high levels of stress, anxiety, and depression regardless of whether the patient lives or dies.[1–4] Family perception of the patient's distress and suffering can also contribute to this. Families are usually called on to be surrogate decision makers for the patient in the ICU, further adding to their burden and emotional needs. The availability of emotional support, information, and appropriate communication for family not only affects their level of distress while in the ICU, but can predict their long-term bereavement and psychosocial outcome and whether or not they develop posttraumatic stress disorder (PTSD), anxiety, or depression.[5,6] How this affects the surviving patient's long-term outcome in turn is not clear, but one can speculate that patient and family distress are interrelated. Standard surgical ICU care must include both interdisciplinary teams and processes of care that specifically address the needs of patients' families with respect to communication, emotional support, information, and decision making.[7,8] If the ICU stay results in the death of the patient, appropriate end-of-life care should also include further support for families in bereavement, decision making, cultural observances, and ample access and time to be at the patient's bedside.

A version of this article was published in the 91:2 issue of *Surgical Clinics of North America*.
[a] Department of Surgery, New Jersey Medical School, University of Medicine and Dentistry of New Jersey, 185 South Orange Avenue, MSB G506, Newark, NJ 07103, USA
[b] Trauma/Critical Care Division, University Hospital - New Jersey Medical School, 150 Bergen Street, Mezz 233, Newark, NJ 07103, USA
* Corresponding author.
*E-mail address:* mosentac@umdnj.edu

Anesthesiology Clin 30 (2012) 37–46
doi:10.1016/j.anclin.2011.11.003       **anesthesiology.theclinics.com**
1932-2275/12/$ – see front matter © 2012 Elsevier Inc. All rights reserved.

## THE FAMILY EXPERIENCE IN THE SICU: GRIEF AND BEREAVEMENT

Grief is a normal but profound emotional reaction to the loss of a loved one. Grief includes diverse emotional, behavioral, cognitive, and physiologic manifestations (**Box 1**). Families may manifest grief in some or all of these ways, at different times, and with different intensity. How families cope with grief will affect their behavior and interactions with the ICU team and the patient. More importantly, how the SICU team supports and interacts with families will have a profound impact on both their acute and long-term bereavement. Grief occurs not only after death, but after any major loss. Even if the patient survives the SICU stay, but has permanent disability, grief may complicate both the patient's and family's recovery. Medical events such as anoxic brain injury, stroke, amputation, or spinal cord injury leading to permanent loss of function mean loss of hopes, expectations, and life as previously known. Such a situation can be devastating—families and patients will experience the same sequence of grief and coping mechanisms as is apparent after a death.

---

**Box 1**
**Manifestations of grief**

*Emotional*
- Despair
- Anxiety
- Guilt
- Anger
- Hostility
- Loneliness

*Behavioral*
- Agitation
- Fatigue
- Crying
- Social withdrawal

*Cognitive*
- Decreased self-esteem
- Preoccupation with the image of deceased
- Helplessness
- Hopelessness
- Self-blame
- Problems with concentration

*Physiologic*
- Anorexia
- Sleep disturbances
- Energy loss and exhaustion
- Somatic complaints
- Susceptibility to illness/disease

In a surgical or trauma ICU the family may be facing the death of a loved one suddenly and without warning, while in other cases the critical illness may follow a long period of chronic illness and disability with significant stress on families as care-givers even before the ICU admission. If the ICU admission follows a transplant or oncologic surgery, families may have high hopes and expectation for life-changing surgery and "rescue." If these hopes are not met, families have difficulty coping with this reality, and may be further overwhelmed. Even if patients die after weeks or months of a long illness, to families this is still a sudden and acutely disruptive event. Their experience of the ICU stay, while "routine" for the staff, may be one of turbu-lence, uncertainty, and hope alternating with despair, all depending on the condition of the patient; families become exhausted, ignoring their own needs for rest and food. Families have probably coped with emotional distress and impending loss using the defense of denial. Death of the patient now shatters that defense. In all of these scenarios grief will be manifest as anger, denial, blame, anxiety, and sorrow.

The ability of families to cope with grief is affected by the social and cultural context in which they live, the nature and availability of support systems,[9] previous loss, and their coping styles. Sudden death or death related to trauma or violence may compli-cate the ability to cope. Increasing evidence suggests that death in the ICU is experi-enced as traumatic for many families, and their bereavement is complicated in a similar way, if they are not supported.[1,4,10,11] Grief and bereavement theory suggests several reasons for this that are relevant to care of families in the SICU (**Box 2**).

## FAMILY AS SURROGATE DECISION MAKER

Twenty percent of patient deaths in the United States occur in the ICU.[12] Ninety percent of deaths in the ICU occur after decisions to withhold or withdraw life-sustaining treatments; however, fewer than 5% of ICU patients have sufficient capacity to make their own decisions about care.[13] Only 10% of ICU patients have advance directives, though advance directives may still not clearly elucidate the nuances of which plan of care would be desired by the patient.[14] These difficult deci-sions regarding treatment limitation and life support are left to be made by surro-gates—the patients' families. Families already under stress due to grief and emotional distress may be further stressed when asked to be the surrogate decision makers; this can interfere with patient care and medical decision making, depending on the ability of families to cope. Complicated grief of the family can lead to conflict

---

**Box 2**
**Experiences of grief by patient families in the SICU**

- The shock of the death overwhelms the self and diminishes ability to cope.
- The perception of the world as orderly and meaningful is shattered, leading to intense reactions of fear, anxiety, and loss of control.
- The mourner experiences a profound loss of security and confidence in the world causing increased anxiety.
- The loss does not make sense and cannot be absorbed.
- There is no chance to say goodbye, leaving unfinished business with the deceased.
- Families have a strong need to determine blame and affix responsibility for it.
- The loss highlights events around the time of death, distorting recollections of the relationship with the deceased and causing survivor guilt.

within families or with the medical team, prolonging end-of-life care and undermining decision making for the patient. Conversely, when stressed families are asked to understand sophisticated medical information and make life and death decisions for another, the role of surrogate not only becomes an unwanted burden, but compounds their own grief and distress. Their ability to cope with grief and bereavement can become further impaired, just when the patient's care needs them most. One-third to one-half of families show signs of depression, anxiety, and posttraumatic stress symptoms while their loved one is in the ICU.[1,3,4,10] These emotional factors are more apparent if the patient dies, but are most heightened if the families have participated in end-of-life decision making as a surrogate, or have experienced discordance or conflict in their decision-making role.[3,4,15] Several studies followed families after ICU discharge. Forty-two percent of families of ICU patients experienced significant anxiety, 16% experienced depression, and 35% had PTSD at 6 months after a loved one's death.[1] Family mental health scores in health-related quality of life assessments were impaired at 90 days after patient discharge; this was associated with end-of-life treatment limitation decisions as well as perceived conflict around care.[16] Families may confuse their involvement as surrogate decision makers, and believe that they are solely responsible for making life and death decisions. The presence of an advance directive, or a previous conversation with the patient about their preferences for treatment, can alleviate some of this burden for families. Although it has been shown that as they are currently used, advance directives do not affect the cost of ICU care and do not change ICU end-of-life decision making,[17] they are effective tools to guide both families and physicians and diminish long-term feelings of guilt, complicated grief, and distress.

While the family's role as surrogate is affected by grief and emotional stress, it can also be affected by their social and cultural community, life circumstances, and coping styles. The expectation in Western medicine that patient autonomy is the prevailing ethical principle may add additional stress to family members from cultures where elders, religious leaders, or male relatives would normally make important decisions. Sociologic study has revealed factors that can support or detract from family ability to function as a surrogate (**Table 1**).[18]

How families cope as surrogate decision makers is also affected by their perception of the critical illness and prognosis of the patient's condition. Families may not rely

**Table 1**
**Family social factors that affect role as surrogate**

| Helps | Hinders |
| --- | --- |
| Previous experiences as decision makers | Competing responsibilities in family |
| Presence of coping skills | Surrogate's poor health |
| Religious support<br>Decisions that align with surrogate beliefs | Financial burdens |
| Support in friend/family network<br>Sense of keeping a patient promise | Family conflicts |
| Sense that decision helps the patient (ie, avoid suffering)<br>Feeling involved in patient care | Personal attachment to patient |
| Knowing patient preferences | Not knowing patient preferences |

*Adapted from* Vig EK, Starks HS, Taylor JS, et al. Surviving surrogate decision-making: what helps and hampers the experience of making medical decisions for others. J Gen Intern Med 2007;22:1274–9.

solely on physician prognostications or medical information in forming their opinions on the loved one's condition or chances for recovery. While in some cases this may reflect a lack of trust in the medical system, it is equally likely that it reflects beliefs about the patient's character, strength of will ("he's a fighter"), belief in miracles, or religious faith.[19] When asked to discuss a patient's chance of survival, both the critically ill and their surrogates predict a higher chance of survival then their actual survival rate or APACHE II predicted mortality.[20] There was no difference in families' understanding of prognostication or incorporation into goal setting if told prognostic information in numerical terms (ie, "Your father has a 10% chance of survival") versus descriptive terms (ie, "Your father is seriously ill"). In addition, after being told in these specific terms about likelihood of death, a patient's surrogate still perceived the chance of survival as higher than the physician's estimate.[21] Families' perception of illness among the critically ill is more influenced by their own emotional and cognitive beliefs—faith, sense of personal control, belief in success/failure of medical therapy— than by prognostications of physicians.[22,23] These perceptions, in turn, clearly will affect a family's ability to set appropriate goals of care and treatment plans for the patient. Key elements of their conceptualization and beliefs are described in **Box 3**.

A recent study suggests that when soliciting reactions to the aforementioned domains from patients and surrogates about their critical illness state, there are differences in perception between groups. African Americans were more likely to be optimistic about the illness but also felt they had less understanding of the disease when compared with Caucasians. In addition, the presence of Christian faith or activity in church was an independent predictor of belief that medical treatment would improve the illness course. African Americans and those patients who identify a strong faith or participation in church are two groups who are more likely to pursue aggressive care and are reluctant to withdraw life support.[24,25] Though not definitively shown, it is possible this treatment preference is related to perceptions about disease. While this remains an area for further study, we must acknowledge that the surrogate's perception of the patient's situation is influenced not only by medical facts but also by family beliefs and background regarding medical information.

## WHAT DO FAMILIES NEED?

Much of the emotional and spiritual suffering around the end of life in the SICU is experienced by the family. Studies on breaking bad news after sudden death have shown that the manner in which death or poor outcome is relayed to the family can have lifelong ramifications for their bereavement.[26] A survey of surviving families of trauma

---

**Box 3**
**Family factors affecting perception of illness and prognosis**

- Chronologic course of illness (acute vs chronic)
- Likely outcome of illness
- Emotional impact of illness
- Sense of personal control over illness state
- Ability of medical care to improve illness state
- Perception of personal understanding

*Data from* Ford D, Zapka J, Gebregziabher M, et al. Factors associated with illness perception among critically ill patients and surrogates. Chest 2010;138:59–67.

patients notes that the top 3 things they value in the care of their loved ones were a caring attitude of the news giver, the clarity of the message, and the opportunity to ask questions.[27] Family needs are more complex when death and dying occurs in the setting of treatment limitation options and surrogate decisions. Several studies have identified factors that positively affect surrogate decision-maker experience, and minimize family stress and iatrogenic suffering **Box 4**.[18]

Studies show that there are specific interventions that can positively affect the care of dying patients' families. The positive impact of hospital-based bereavement services, pastoral care, or family support personnel is becoming increasingly apparent on the long-term psychosocial functioning of surviving families and on other outcomes, such as organ donation.[28,29] Many interventions revolve around establishing a communication plan, providing written materials about the patient's condition, addressing end-of-life care early, and providing bereavement and emotional support. ICUs that have standard processes of care such as a "communication bundle" (ie, family meetings within 72 hours, emotional support within 24 hours) have a positive impact on family outcomes.[7,8] Setting up an intensive communication plan aimed at families, which provides emotional, educational, and decisional support, will establish therapeutic goals based on patient preferences *earlier*, decrease conflict, and decrease family distress, without a significant change in patient mortality.[30–34] In addition, family leaflets providing information regarding disease and treatment have been shown to improve comprehension and satisfaction among families with the capability to understand the medical care.[5,6] Finally, initiating discussion of end-of-life care both as education and support before decisions need to be made has been shown to alleviate stress, anxiety, and depression regarding these issues. Talking about end-of-life issues early provides families with a structured forum to expose their individual needs

---

**Box 4**
**Factors affecting family distress as surrogate decision makers**

*Decrease Distress*

- Unlimited access to loved ones
- Family meetings, sense of clinician availability
- Privacy
- Communication involving a show of compassion, respect, listening, and honesty
- Hope, dignity, choice, and finding meaning in patient experience
- Patient comfort and free of suffering
- Frank information about condition and prognosis from clinicians
- Recommendations from clinicians
- Support for surrogate choices from clinicians

*Increase Distress*

- Lack of clear data or contradictory information
- Infrequent discussions or discussion in a busy place (ie, waiting room)
- Conflicts between team members

*Data from* Vig EK, Starks HS, Taylor JS, et al. Surviving surrogate decision-making: what helps and hampers the experience of making medical decisions for others. J Gen Intern Med 2007;22:1274–9.

and concerns, as well as express any guilt they may have regarding being involved in end-of-life decision making.[26,32]

## PALLIATIVE CARE INTERVENTIONS TO SUPPORT FAMILIES IN THE ICU

To support families in the ICU both for bereavement and as surrogate decision makers requires systematic processes of care as well as an interdisciplinary team. Family satisfaction and long-term bereavement outcomes are improved with communication and emotional support interventions.[5,6,27,28,32,33] There are several keys to understanding the approach to successful family communication in the ICU setting. First, it is important to recognize communication as a defined process and skill with specific approaches to improve family satisfaction.[33,35] Just as there are a series of key steps

---

**Box 5**
**SPIKES: A 6-step protocol for delivering bad news**

*Step 1: S: Setting up the interview*
- Arrange for privacy and a quiet place
- Involve key family members
- Sit down and introduce yourself
- Make connection with the family
- Manage time constraints and interruptions

*Step 2: P: assessing the family's Perception*
- Find out what the family already knows

*Step 3: I: obtaining the family's Invitation*
- Find out what the family wants to know

*Step 4: K: giving Knowledge and information to the family*
- Avoid medical jargon
- Give information in small amounts at a time
- Educate about patient's condition and prognosis
- Express uncertainty honestly

*Step 5: E: addressing the family's Emotions with Empathetic responses*
- Listen and respond to family's feelings
- Allow time for expression of emotion
- Identify family's emotion
- Identify cause of emotion
- Connect emotion with the cause of emotion

*Step 6: S: Strategy and Summary*
- Discuss goals of care
- Treatment plans
- Future meetings

*From* Buckman R. Communication in palliative care: a practical guide. In: Doyle D, Hanks GWC, McDonald N, editors. Oxford textbook of palliative medicine. 2nd edition. New York: Oxford University Press; 1998; p. 141–56; with permission.

---

for any procedure or algorithm, preparation is required for successful family communication. Second, families' readiness to accept bad news and their response to grief is also a process and takes time. While the patient in the ICU may be critically ill and need immediate decisions to be made about the next step in care, families must be ready and willing to undertake the task of becoming decision makers, and this cannot be rushed despite the acuity of the patient's situation. It takes time to build a trusting and collaborative relationship with a patient's family. Several communication approaches that improve family satisfaction and outcomes have been well described.[32,35,36] The SPIKES protocol and the VALUE protocol are two examples. Buckman[36] outlined 6 steps to communicate bad news to patients' loved ones, and an adaptation for families is shown in **Box 5**.

Interdisciplinary communication both educates and supports the family. The whole ICU team should be involved in this process to prevent iatrogenic suffering of the family as much as possible. Several models of interdisciplinary communication have been shown to be effective as emotional and decisional support for families, especially in their role as surrogate decision maker.[4–6,30,31,34,37] The team should include the physician, the nurse, a psychosocial or bereavement support professional, and spiritual/pastoral care. While physicians provide expertise in medical information and prognosis, others can support the family particularly in their role as surrogate. Each member of the team has a different role, but many may have direct contact with patients and their families. Every member is a potential resource to a patient's family. Consensus among all caregivers is important not only for cohesive patient care but also for family care; families identify conflict within the medical team as one of the distressing aspects of care in the ICU.[18] Critical care nurses have wide exposure to a patient's loved ones. Families appear to receive important communication through nurses and rate their skill in communication as one of the more important in their experience.[38] Although nurses often have more access to patients' families and by the nature of that exposure are a key element of communication regarding patient care, there are data to suggest they are not inherently better at this communication than doctors.[39] This problem can be addressed by bringing all members of the team up to speed on patient prognosis and care goals during morning rounds or in a structured format. Nurses may benefit from training to specifically improve their communication skills.

## REFERENCES

1. Anderson WG, Arnold RM, Angus DC, et al. Posttraumatic stress and complicated grief in family members of patients in the intensive care unit. J Gen Intern Med 2008;23(11):1871–6.
2. McAdam JL, Dracup KA, White DB, et al. Symptom experiences of families of intensive care unit patients. Crit Care Med 2010;38:1075–85.
3. Pochard F, Darmon M, Fassier T, et al. Symptoms of anxiety and depression in family members of intensive care unit patients before discharge or death. a prospective multicenter study. J Crit Care 2005;20:90–6.
4. Azoulay E, Pochard F, Kentish-Barnes N, et al. Risk of post-traumatic stress symptoms in family members of intensive care unit patients. Am J Respir Crit Care Med 2005;171:987–94.
5. Azoulay E, Pochard F, Chevret S, et al. Impact of a family information leaflet on effectiveness of information provided to family members of intensive care unit patients: a multicentre, prospective, randomized, controlled trail. Am J Respir Crit Care Med 2002;165:438–42.

6. Lautrette A, Darmon M, Megarbane B, et al. A communication strategy and brochure for relatives of patients dying in the ICU. N Engl J Med 2007;356: 469–78.
7. Nelson JE, Brasel KJ, Campbell ML, et al. for the IPAL_ICU Project. Evaluation of ICU palliative care quality: a technical assistance monograph from the IPAL-ICU Project. Center to Advance Palliative Care 2010. [Epub ahead of print].
8. Robert D, Truog MA, Margaret L, et al. Recommendations for end-of-life care in the intensive care unit: a consensus statement by the American Academy of Critical Care Medicine. Crit Care Med 2008;36(3):953–63.
9. Rando T. Treatment of complicated mourning. Champaign (IL): Research Press; 1993.
10. Siegel M, Hayes E, Vandereweker L, et al. Psychiatric illness in the next of kin of patients who die in the ICU. Crit Care Med 2008;36:1722–5.
11. Van der Klink MA, Heijboer L, Hofhuis JG, et al. Survey into bereavement of family members of patients who died in the intensive care unit. Intensive Crit Care Nurs 2010;26:215–25.
12. Linde-Zwirble W, Angus DC, Griffin M, et al. ICU care at the end-of-life in America: an epidemiological study. Crit Care Med 2000;28:A34.
13. Prendergast TJ, Luce JM. Increasing incidence of withholding and withdrawal of life support from the critically ill. Am J Respir Crit Care Med 1997;155: 15–20.
14. Danis M, Mutran E, Garrett JM, et al. A prospective study of the impact of patient preferences on life-sustaining treatment and hospital cost. Crit Care Med 1996; 24:1811–7.
15. Gries CJ, Engelberg RA, Kross EK, et al. Predictors of symptoms of posttraumatic stress and depression in family members after patient death in the ICU. Chest 2010;137:280–7.
16. Lemiale V, Kentish-Barnes N, Chaize M, et al. Health-related quality of life in family members of intensive care unit patients. J Palliat Med 2010;13:1131–7.
17. Teno JM, Lynn J, Wenger N, et al. Advance directives for seriously ill hospitalized patients: effectiveness with the patient self-determination act and the SUPPORT intervention. SUPPORT Investigators. Study to understand prognoses and preferences for outcomes and risks of treatment. J Am Geriatr Soc 1997;45:500–70.
18. Vig EK, Starks HS, Taylor JS, et al. Surviving surrogate decision-making: what helps and hampers the experience of making medical decisions for others. J Gen Intern Med 2007;22:1274–9.
19. Boyd EA, Lo B, Evans LR, et al. "Its not just what the doctor tells me" factors that influences surrogate decision-makers' perceptions of prognosis. Crit Care Med 2010;38:1270–5.
20. Ford D, Zapka JG, Gebregziabher M, et al. Investigating critically ill patients' and families' perceptions of likelihood of survival. J Palliat Med 2009;12(1):45–52.
21. Lee Char SJ, Evans LR, Malvar GL, et al. A randomized trial of two methods to disclose prognosis to surrogate decision makers in intensive care units. Am J Respir Crit Care Med 2010;182(7):905–9.
22. Ford D, Zapka J, Gebregziabher M, et al. Factors associated with illness perception among critically ill patients and surrogates. Chest 2010;138:59–67.
23. Leventhal H, Meyer D, Nerenz DR. The common-sense representation of illness danger. In: Rachman S, editor. Medical psychology. New York: Pergamon; 1980. p. 7–30.
24. Hopp FP, Duffy SA. Racial variations in end-of-life-care. J Am Geriatr Soc 2000; 48:658–63.

25. Phelps AC, Maciejewski PK, Nilsson M, et al. Religious coping and use of intensive life-prolonging care near death in patients with advanced cancer. JAMA 2009;301:1140–7.
26. Iverson K. Grave words: notifying survivors about sudden unexpected deaths. Tucson (AZ): Galen Press; 1999.
27. Jurkevich GJ, Pierce B, Pananen L, et al. Giving bad news: the family perspective. J Trauma 2000;48:865–73.
28. Oliver RD, Sturtevant JP, Scheetz JP, et al. Beneficial effects of a hospital bereavement intervention program after traumatic childhood death. J Trauma 2001;50:440–8.
29. Linyear AS, Tartaglia A. Family communication coordination: a program to increase organ donation. J Transpl Coord 1999;9:165–74.
30. Lilly CM, De Meo DL, Sonna LA, et al. An intensive communication intervention for the critically ill. Am J Med 2000;109:469–75.
31. Mosenthal AC, Murphy PA, Barker LK, et al. Changing the culture of end of life care in the trauma ICU. J Trauma 2008;64(6):1587–93.
32. Curtis JR, Patrick DL, Shannon SE, et al. The family conference as a focus to improve communication about end-of-life care in the intensive care unit: opportunities for improvement. Crit Care Med 2001;29(Suppl 2):N26–33.
33. Curtis JR, Engelberg RA, Wenrich MD, et al. Missed opportunities during family conferences about end-of-life care in the intensive care unit. Am J Respir Crit Care Med 2005;171:844–9.
34. Schneiderman LJ, Gilmer T, Teetzel HD, et al. Effect of ethics consultations on nonbeneficial life-sustaining treatments in the intensive care setting: a randomized controlled trial. JAMA 2003;290:1166–72.
35. Stapleton RD, Engelberg RA, Wenrich MD, et al. Clinician statements and family satisfaction with family conferences in the intensive care unit. Crit Care Med 2006; 34:1679–85.
36. Buckman R. Communication in palliative care: a practical guide. In: Dereck D, editor. Oxford textbook of palliative medicine. 2nd edition. Oxford (England): Oxford University Press; 1998. p. 141–58.
37. Mcdonagh JR, Elliott TB, Engelberg RA, et al. Family satisfaction with family conferences about end of life care in the intensive care unit: increased proportion of family speech is associated with increased satisfaction. Crit Care Med 2004; 32:1484–8.
38. Hickey M. What are the needs of families of critically ill patients? A review of the literature since 1976. Heart Lung 1990;19:401–15.
39. Maguire PA, Faulkner A. Helping cancer patients disclose their concerns. Eur J Cancer 1996;32:78–81.

# Communication as a Core Skill of Palliative Surgical Care

Thomas J. Miner, MD

KEYWORDS

• Surgical palliation • Palliative triangle • Communication skills

*The skill and effort that we put into our clinical communication does make an indelible impression on our patients, their families, and their friends. If we do it badly, they may never forgive us; if we do it well, they may never forget us.*
— *Robert Buckman*[1]

Surgeons, by necessity, manage a broad spectrum of death and dying. Death can occur unexpectedly in the otherwise healthy individual because of an unexpected trauma, an unidentified medical condition, such as a ruptured aortic aneurysm, or a catastrophic perioperative event. A patient with severe burns or multiple organ failure in the intensive care unit may die after a period of prolonged uncertainty about possible recovery. Patients with chronic disease also die quite expectedly. Surgeons commonly care for and operate on such patients. Given the nature of perioperative practice, a broad expertise in communicating with patients and their families about these difficult circumstances is required.

The public and those in the medical profession are increasingly concerned about the adequacy and suitability of end-of-life care. Therapy aimed at prolonging life with little attention to relieving patient suffering has resulted in an increasing demand for placing quality of life over quantity of life. Government involvement and public discussions of death and dying often include debates about euthanasia and physician-assisted suicide, a move toward advance directives, and the need for improved hospice care.[2–5] Although comprehensive end-of-life care has been identified as the standard of care for dying patients, this care is widely recognized to be deficient.[6,7] Recent initiatives in palliative medicine, the therapeutic goals of which emphasize support and symptom management, are attempting to improve this critical aspect of the total care of patients with cancer.

A version of this article was published in the 91:2 Issue of *Surgical Clinics of North America*.
Department of Surgery, The Alpert Medical School of Brown University, Rhode Island Hospital, 593 Eddy Street, APC 4, Providence, RI 02903, USA
*E-mail address:* TMiner@USASURG.org

Anesthesiology Clin 30 (2012) 47–58
doi:10.1016/j.anclin.2011.11.004                                    anesthesiology.theclinics.com
1932-2275/12/$ – see front matter © 2012 Elsevier Inc. All rights reserved.

Being in twenty-first century, we confront a timeless and inescapable certainty of the human condition: that death is a natural fact of life.[8] About 50 years ago, it was common for physicians, patients, and families to avoid discussing cancer diagnoses. Conversations regarding diagnoses, treatment options, and prognoses, now take place routinely, and open disclosure has become a core principal of good clinical practice.[9] However, appropriate communication between patients and physicians is still lacking. In a recent study, more than 20% of patients were told their cancer diagnosis in an impersonal manner, suggesting that many physicians are either unacquainted with or unskilled at good communication. In a significant number of patients this communication in an impersonal manner was associated with a lack of trust or a bad relationship with the physician and was cited as a reason for changing physicians.[9] The high expectations of the general public and patients demand an effective use of communication skills to permit active participation in their health care decisions. At the end of life, patients and families seek well-developed communication and interpersonal skills to guide them during this particularly vulnerable time.[10] These high expectations fall on all of those who care for end of life patients, including surgeons, anesthesiologists, internists, physician extenders (nurse practitioners or physician's assistants), and nursing professionals.

## SURGICAL PALLIATION

For decades, surgeons have been at the forefront in the movement toward palliative care. The roots of many current operations and operations used until recently to achieve a surgical "cure" can be traced back to procedures designed to alleviate symptomatic and often painful disease. In 1882, William Halstead introduced radical mastectomy to manage the pain emanating from locally advanced and ulcerating breast cancer, but this procedure was also found to be effective in sometimes curing cancer.[11] Similarly, coronary artery bypass grafting was first advocated for the symptomatic relief of angina pectoris but was then found to have survival benefits.[12] Many surgeons are not prepared to effectively administer palliative care despite a clear and well-established role. Surgical training in palliation is cursory, there is not enough quantity and quality of peer-reviewed literature,[4] and surgical textbooks[13] are generally lacking. This shortage of training and literature might explain why surgeons traditionally have been poor at communicating with patients about end-of-life issues.[14]

Palliative care has been defined by the World Health Organization[15] as "the total active care of patients whose disease is not responsive to curative treatment. Control of pain, of other symptoms, and of psychological, social, and spiritual problems, is paramount. The goal of palliative care is achievement of the best quality of life for patients and their families." Others have further defined surgical palliation to include (1) initial evaluation of the disease, (2) local control of the disease, (3) control of discharge or hemorrhage, (4) control of pain, and (5) reconstruction and rehabilitation. Although these broad definitions provide a global understanding of the reaches of palliative care, alternate interpretations of what constitutes a palliative surgical procedure by different clinicians and investigators render comparisons between and, at times, within studies problematic. Because ideal palliative care requires an approach defined in terms of the patient's individual needs and values, identical procedures may play dramatically different roles for each patient. Identifying surgical palliation by the type of procedure performed, rather than by the goals and intentions of the procedure, is of limited value. Designation of procedures as palliative based on the extent of disease (ranging from gross disease at operation to postoperative margin status) rather than on a sound understanding of the elements associated with good palliative therapy is equally fruitless. Surgical palliation is best defined as the deliberate use of a procedure in a patient with incurable disease with the intention of relieving symptoms, minimizing patient distress, and improving quality of life. Palliation is not the opposite of cure. Each term has its own distinct indications and goals that should be evaluated independently. By defining palliation based on factors such as symptom control and surgical intent, the primary focus on an individualized approach for palliative surgery is maintained. An association between palliative intent and surgical outcomes has been well demonstrated in patients with cancer in the literature. The effectiveness of a palliative intervention should be judged by the presence and durability of patient-acknowledged symptom resolution. During the palliative phase of care, endeavors to improve the overall survival should not outweigh the efforts aimed at minimizing the morbidity, mortality, or duration of treatment. Although symptom palliation may result in increased survival for the individual patient, it is inappropriate to select a palliative procedure based solely on a desire for improved duration of survival.[16–20]

Palliation of complications from advanced cancer demands the highest level of surgical judgment and serves as an excellent model for considering surgical palliation. Although surgical issues for cancer sites can differ, the indications for surgical palliative procedures generally fall into 3 main areas of concern: obstruction, bleeding, and perforation. Individual patients also may present with more chronic complaints such as pain, nausea, vomiting, inability to eat, anemia, or jaundice. When considering the appropriate and effective use of palliative procedures, a surgeon is often confronted with a full range of multidisciplinary treatment options and technical considerations that could potentially relieve some of the symptoms of an advanced malignancy. Practitioners must often deliberate over options that are outside their individual experience. Although consideration of risk in terms of treatment-related toxicity, morbidity, and mortality is an important part of the surgical decision-making process, attention to this element should not be the sole factor in making decisions about palliative therapy. Decisions are best made on end points such as the probability of symptom resolution, the effect on overall quality of life, pain control, and cost effectiveness. Regardless of the anatomic site and cause leading to the need for palliative intervention, deliberations over surgical palliation must consider the medical condition and performance status of the patient, the natural history of the primary and secondary symptoms, the extent and prognosis of the cancer, the potential success and durability of the procedure, the availability and success of nonsurgical management, and the individual patient's quality and expectancy of life. Owing to the significant morbidity and mortality associated with palliative procedures, the single most important factor demonstrated in the literature in successful palliation is clearly proper patient selection. Because of the limited research and predominately anecdotal experience in this field, treatment algorithms and well-established surgical dictums are essentially nonexistent. However, from the largest prospective trial to date, it is known that poor performance status, poor nutrition, and no previous cancer therapy are factors that indicate patients who will do poorly.[20] Through the palliative phase of a patient's disease, specific complaints may change and goals may be redefined many times. Therapy for symptoms must remain flexible and individualized to meet continually the patient's unique and ever-changing needs. This is a situation in which surgical judgment is imperative, because these problems cannot be thought of in terms of right or wrong.[21]

Optimal palliative decision making is facilitated through effective interactions and direct communication between the patient, family members, and the surgeon through an indomitable relationship described as palliative triangle (**Fig. 1**). Through the dynamics of the triangle, the patient's complaints, values, and emotional support

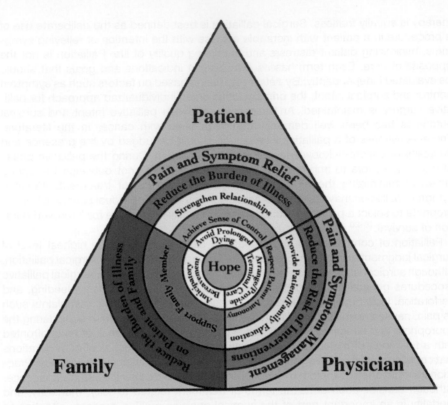

**Fig. 1.** The palliative triangle. Interactions between the patient, the family, and the surgeon guide individual decisions regarding palliative care. The hope for potentially achievable goals is advanced as each participant of the palliative triangle fulfills specific obligations. Good communication between the patient, the family, and the surgeon is essential for the palliative triangle to be effective. (*From* Thomay AA, Jaques DP, Miner TJ. Surgical palliation: getting back to our roots. Surg Clin North Am 2009;89:33; with permission.)

are considered against the known medical and surgical alternatives. Outcomes data obtained through reports on surgical palliation can be especially useful to submit accurate information regarding chance of success, procedure-related durability, the possibility for complications, and anticipated survival. Another important factor is anticipating, understanding, and addressing a patient's and/or a family's expectations about the intent of the proposed procedure. The palliative intent needs to be understood and explicitly agreed upon. Although patients, family members, and surgeons may at times have incongruent expectations, the dynamics of the palliative triangle help to moderate such beliefs and guide the decision-making process toward the best possible choice for the patient. This strong relationship may also explain the observation of high patient satisfaction toward surgeons after palliative operations, even in patients having no demonstrable benefit from surgery or in those experiencing serious complications. Patients are satisfied because the surgeon was there for them at this difficult time of great need; discussed the risks, benefits, and alternatives of all of their choices; and remained engaged with them throughout the remainder of their lives.[14,16]

Even though the thoughtfulness, judgment, and time required to make such complicated palliative decisions are appreciated by patients and families, some physicians and surgeons shy away from this process with the explanation that they do not want to take away hope from those battling cancer. Cleary, it is inappropriate to suggestprolonged survival to be provided by an operation performed with a palliative intent. Rather than focusing on what cannot be provided (cure), emphasis must be placed on those things that can be realistically delivered. As the palliative triangle suggests, a successful palliative surgeon places this definition of hope at the center of a patient's overall care. It is rational for the patient with advanced cancer to hope for quality of life, symptom resolution, technically superior palliative operations, dignity, and compassion. Through continued personal interactions and deliberate communication, each participant of the palliative triangle contributes to making a unique patient-centered decision, recognizing that varying procedures will have different goals for every individual. Although identical procedures can be performed for similar clinical problems, whether it is right of wrong depends on the unique circumstances of each patient.[14]

The discipline has evolved to recognize that palliative surgical treatment options are not right for every patient and that care must be individualized in a multidisciplinary manner that is most appropriate for a specific patient. There will be times when the most appropriate decision a surgeon can make in the treatment of a terminally ill patient is not to perform an operation. However, this means that a surgeon will have to say "no" to a significant number of patients, who are thought to possess too much risk without a reasonable expectation of benefit. Surgeons must be cautious never to promise an outcome that they cannot realistically expect to deliver. When recognizing those patients who are at risk for procedure-related complications or death or those in whom a particular procedure is unlikely to provide an idealized benefit, surgeons should understand that saying "no" is appropriate. If communicated effectively, the patient will ultimately understand that this response does not represent abandonment or failure on the part of the surgeon but rather a team approach to minimizing symptoms without sacrificing quality of life.[14]

## COMMUNICATORS IN THE PERIOPERATIVE PERIOD

Effective use of communication skills by physicians benefits both the physician and the patient and is a key element of a successful therapeutic relationship. Physicians' communication skills are associated with important patient and physician outcomes.[22,23] These outcomes include physician and patient satisfaction,[24,25] patient participation in care and adjustment to illness,[26] malpractice liability,[27] and important clinical markers of health.[28–31] When doctors communicate well with their patients, clinical problems are identified more accurately, patients are more satisfied with their care, treatment plans are more likely to be followed, feelings of distress and vulnerability are lessened, and physicians' well-being is improved.[32] Back and colleagues[33] argue that although physicians often learn good interviewing skills, their training does not promote proficiency in second-order communication skills, such as conveying empathy and understanding. This lack of training complicates situations in which bad or difficult news is commonly discussed. Some find that their lack of training or discomfort with emotionally charged negative information at times leads to unpleasant interactions.[34]

The importance of good communication skills in surgical practice is undeniable.[10] One study comparing primary care physicians with surgeons showed that surgeons spend more time emphasizing patient education and counseling.[35] Surgeons deliver bad news frequently in the course of their careers.[36] Surgeons are confronted, not uncommonly, with other challenging experiences such as requesting permission for autopsy or organ donation.[23] Because surgeons frequently deal with gravely sick and dying patients, surveyed surgeons have identified breaking bad news and bereavement counseling as areas worthy of instruction for surgical trainees.[37]

Competence in palliative care requires not only sound clinical decision making but also skill in communication and building relationships. Although communication barriers may involve the patient and family, or even the health system itself, the surgeon bears the major responsibility for conducting the communications well.[38] Communication is often the most important component of palliative care, and effective symptom control is virtually impossible without effective communication.[39] In addition to the fact that communication provides the structure and context of good surgical palliative decisions, it is sometimes all that can be offered. Compared with other palliative therapies, communication skills have clear palliative efficacy (reduces patient anxiety and distress) and a wide therapeutic index (treatment-related morbidity and mortality is rare), and their most common problem in practice is suboptimal dosing.[1]

Most practitioners are not trained in effective communication techniques during the perioperative period, and many are left to learn by trial and error and frequently miss empathic opportunities.[40] Although some through practice, intuition, or study are highly skilled at delivering bad news and at negotiating patients' reactions to bad news empathically, many are not as effective communicators as they think they are or should be.[34] An effort to improve surgical palliative care in the future will require the thoughtful education of future and current surgeons not only in sound palliative decision making but also in communication skills. With the restrictions to residency training secondary to managed care and work hour regulations, surgical training programs have increasingly become algorithm based. Although this transformation likely works with the old surgical adage of "see one, do one, teach one," all too often, residents looking for guidance in the proper conversations of palliative care never get the opportunity to "see one." Robert Milch summed up this idea best in his talk on palliative care in surgical resident education at the American College of Surgeons Clinical Congress in 2003 as, "if you think about it, demonstration of competency in communication skills is much like performing an operation. We would never think of sending an untutored, un-mentored, unsupervised house officer into an operating room to do a procedure never seen, modeled, or performed before, and about which he had only read in a book. Yet this sort of demand for communication skills is one on which we place our house officers all the time, and they have not been taught good communication skills. And very often they have not seen it modeled or mentored."[41]

Although there are several programs to improve communication skills in surgical trainees, the vast majority of surgical training programs have no set curriculum in which to teach palliative care.[34,42,43] However, in a study from the author's institution, 47 general surgery residents were surveyed, and all thought that managing end-of life issues are valuable skills for a surgeon and that sessions in this topic would be a useful and important part of their training. The study was based on a pilot curriculum in palliative surgical care designed specifically for residents. The curriculum was presented over three 1-hour sessions, and included didactic sessions, group discussions, and role-playing scenarios, and the residents were asked to complete pretest, posttest, and 3-month follow-up surveys. Specific modules to improve communication skill and breaking bad news were included in the workshop. At pretest, only 9% of the residents thought that they had previously received adequate training in palliation during their residency and only 57% stated that they felt comfortable speaking to patients about end-of-life issues. At posttest and 3-month follow-up, however, these goals were met for 85% of the residents. Although this study was not designed for mastery of this complex topic, it demonstrated that surgeons can be introduced effectively to palliative care early in their careers with only a modest time commitment. Residents cited that their biggest problem in interacting with patient and families regarding end-of-life issues was apprehension about dealing with extreme emotional responses. Learning communication techniques to help them navigate effectively through these difficult situations seemed to help trainees overcome this barrier.[44] When used correctly, lessons such as these in conversation and advanced decision making can provide the building block to successful palliation spanning an entire career.[45] Because many efforts such as these to improve communication skills focus on medical students and residents, they often remain isolated in academic settings. The communication skills of the busy surgeon often remain poorly developed, and the need for established physicians to become better communicators continues.[34]

## IMPROVING COMMUNICATION SKILLS

In the 1970s and 1980s, it was widely assumed that communication skills were an innate ability. Coupled with a belief that practitioners should be able to feel or sense what the patient experiences in order to respond intuitively in an appropriate way, many doctors felt alienated to the topic of patient-physician communication because it was excessively "touch-feely." Such a paradigm offers few suggestions or guidelines that could help even highly motivated physicians to improve their skills. In the last 2 to 3 decades, however, researchers have learned that communications skills are acquired skills like any other clinical ability and are not some intangible inherited gift. The knowledge, skills, and behaviors associated with effective communication can be learned and retained with a few techniques applied in a logical sequence.[38,39]

Although there are probably many ways of summarizing and simplifying medical communication, the most practical and popular technique is the context, listening, acknowledgement, strategy, and summary (CLASS) protocol of Buckman.[39] This 5-step basic protocol for medical communication, bearing the acronym CLASS, is easy to remember and use. It also lays a straightforward method for dealing with emotions. The ability to empathize with patients is fundamental to the ultimate success of the exchange but is frequently undervalued because of the disproportionate importance that is placed on reasoning capacity in medical care. As summarized in **Fig. 2**, the CLASS protocol identifies the following 5 main components of medical communication as essential and crucial: context (the physical context or setting), listening skills, acknowledgement of patient's emotions, strategy for clinical management, and summary.[38,39]

The ability to discuss bad news with the patient and family is a clinical skill that is essential for effective communication during end-of-life care. Bad news can be defined as any news that adversely affects patients' view of their future. The goal of skillfully breaking bad news is to reduce the severity and duration of stress and encourage engagement of coping mechanisms, both for physicians and for patients and their caregivers. Learning skills to improve breaking bad news can help to prevent potentially devastating physician interactions leading to the insensitively blunt delivery or "dumping" of bad news to patients and their families. Such occurrences of the "hit and run" delivery of bad news likely result from physicians' own emotional discomfort, perceived lack of time, and insufficient training in empathic communication skills.[34] The setting, patient's perception, invitation, knowledge, emotions, and strategy/summary (SPIKES) protocol (**Fig. 3**), a variant of the basic CLASS approach, has

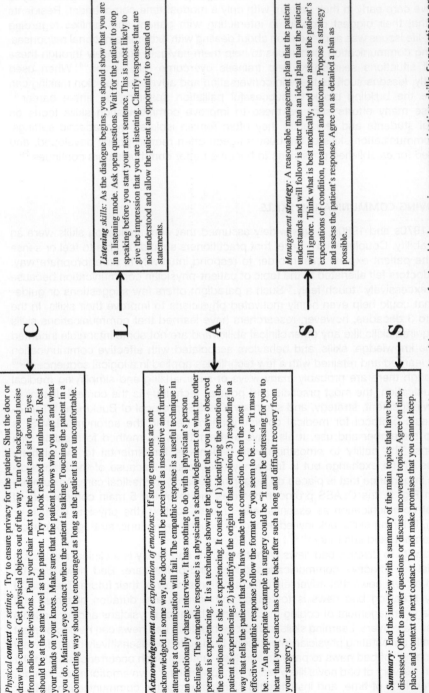

**Fig. 2.** The CLASS protocol. It is a basic method that can be used by any health care professional in improving communication skills. Suggestions on how to implement each element of the protocol are offered. (*Adapted from* Buckman R. Communication skills in palliative care: a practical guide. Neurol Clin 2001;19:989–1004; with permission.)

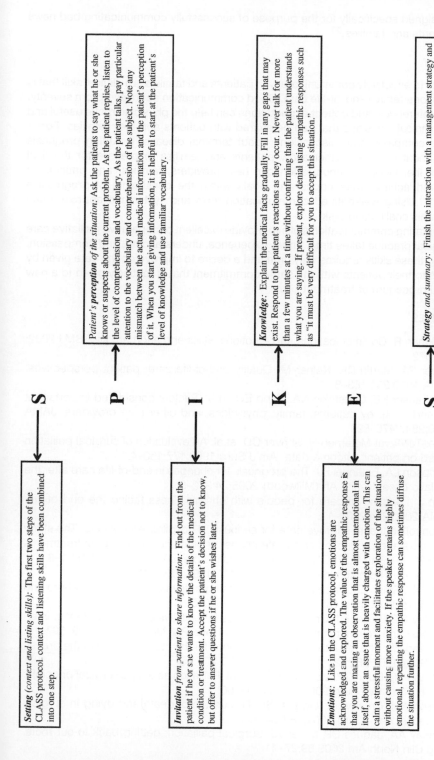

**S**

*Setting (context and listing skills):* The first two steps of the CLASS protocol: context and listening skills have been combined into one step.

**P**

*Patient's perception of the situation:* Ask the patients to say what he or she knows or suspects about the current problem. As the patient replies, listen to the level of comprehension and vocabulary. As the patient talks, pay particular attention to the vocabulary and comprehension of the subject. Note any mismatch between the actual medical information and the patient's perception of it. When you start giving information, it is helpful to start at the patient's level of knowledge and use familiar vocabulary.

**I**

*Invitation from patient to share information:* Find out from the patient if he or she wants to know the details of the medical condition or treatment. Accept the patient's decision not to know, but offer to answer questions if he or she wishes later.

**K**

*Knowledge:* Explain the medical facts gradually. Fill in any gaps that may exist. Respond to the patient's reactions as they occur. Never talk for more than a few minutes at a time without confirming that the patient understands what you are saying. If present, explore denial using empathic responses such as "it must be very difficult for you to accept this situation."

**E**

*Emotions:* Like in the CLASS protocol, emotions are acknowledged and explored. The value of the empathic response is that you are making an observation that is almost unemotional in itself, about an issue that is heavily charged with emotion. This can calm a stressful moment and facilitates exploration of the situation without causing more anxiety. If the speaker remains highly emotional, repeating the empathic response can sometimes diffuse the situation further.

**S**

*Strategy and summary:* Finish the interaction with a management strategy and summary as in the CLASS protocol.

**Fig. 3.** The SPIKES protocol. The listed steps offer a helpful systematic approach of communicating at times when stress is high, such as when delivering bad news. Suggestions on how to implement each element of the protocol are offered. (*Adapted from* Buckman R. Communication skills in palliative care: a practical guide. Neurol Clin 2001;19:989–1004; with permission.)

been designed specifically for the purpose of successfully communicating bad news with patients and families.[39]

## SUMMARY

The ability to effectively communicate with patients and families is a clinical skill that is essential for effective end-of-life care. Good communication about symptom severity, patient preferences, and patient expectations can help the physician make useful and relevant clinical decisions that can be shared with patients and their families. Forthright and compassionate discussions about terminal disease, including prognosis and treatment options, further allow patients and families to prepare for the final stages of life. Good communication can help providers, families, and patients to "clarify and achieve their hopes and goals within the constraints of progressive disease."[46] Using well-defined communication tools and systematic approach can facilitate this challenging task.

Incorporating communication skills to provide excellent perioperative palliative care into surgical practice takes time, effort, experience, understanding, and compassion. Obtaining these skills requires only time and a desire to improve on the care given by surgeons to their patients with the same commitment that is routinely given to a new technical procedure or treatment plan.

## REFERENCES

1. Buckman R. Communications and emotions: skills and effort are key. BMJ 2002; 325:672.
2. Singer PA, Martin DK, Kelner M. Quality end-of-life care: patient perspectives. JAMA 1999;281:163–8.
3. Steinhauser KE, Christakis NA, Clipp EC, et al. Factors considered important at the end of life by patients, family, physicians, and other care providers. JAMA 2000;284:2476–82.
4. Miner TJ, Tavaf-Motamen H, Shriver CD, et al. An evaluation of surgical palliation based on patient outcome data. Am J Surg 1999;177:150–4.
5. Hampson LA, Emanuel EJ. The prognosis for changes in end-of-life care after the Schiavo case. Health Aff (Millwood) 2005;24:972–5.
6. Lynn J. Learning of care for people with chronic illness facing the end of life. JAMA 2000;284:2508–11.
7. A controlled trial to improve care for seriously ill hospitalized patients. The study to understand prognoses and preferences for outcomes and risks of treatments (SUPPORT). The SUPPORT principal investigators. JAMA 2000;274:1591–8.
8. McCue JD. The naturalness of dying. JAMA 1995;273:1039–43.
9. Figg WD, Smith EK, Price DK, et al. Disclosing a diagnosis of cancer: where and how does it occur? J Clin Oncol 2010;28:3630–5.
10. Bradley CT, Brasel KJ. Core competencies in palliative care for surgeons: interpersonal and communications skills. Am J Hosp Pall Med 2008;24:299–507.
11. Halstead WJ. The results of radical operations for the cure of cancer of the breast. Ann Surg 1907;46:1–27.
12. McCahill LE, Dunn GP, Mosenthal AC, et al. Palliation as a core surgical principle: part 1. J Am Coll Surg 2004;199(1):149–60.
13. Easson AM, Crosby JA, Librach SL. Discussion of death and dying in surgical textbooks. Am J Surg 2001;182:34–9.
14. Thomay AA, Jaques DP, Miner TJ. Surgical palliation: getting back to our roots. Surg Clin North Am 2009;89:27–41.

15. World Health Organization. Cancer pain relief and palliative cure: report of a WHO expert committee (technical report series No. 804). Geneva (Switzerland): World Health Organization; 1990. p. 11.
16. Miner TJ, Jaques DP, Shriver CD. A prospective evaluation of patients undergoing surgery for the palliation of an advanced malignancy. Ann Surg Oncol 2002;9:696–703.
17. Miner TJ, Jaques DP, Paty P, et al. Symptom control of locally recurrent rectal cancer. Ann Surg Oncol 2002;10:72–9.
18. Miner TJ, Jaques DP, Karpeh MS, et al. Defining non-curative gastric resections by palliative intent. J Am Coll Surg 2004;198:1013–21.
19. Miner TJ, Karpeh MS. Gastrectomy for gastric cancer: defining critical elements of patient selection and outcome assessment. Surg Oncol Clin N Am 2004;13: 455–66.
20. Miner TJ, Brennan MF, Jaques DP. A prospective, symptom related, outcomes analysis of 1,022 palliative procedures for advanced cancer. Ann Surg 2004; 240:719–27.
21. Miner TJ. Palliative surgery for advanced cancer: lessons learned in patient selection and outcome assessment. Am J Clin Oncol 2005;28:411–4.
22. Makoul G. Essential elements of communication in medical encounters: the Kalamazoo consensus statement. Acad Med 2001;76:390–3.
23. Kalet AL, Janicik R, Schwarz M, et al. Teaching communication skills on the surgery clerkship. Med Educ Online 2005;10:1–7.
24. Levinson W, Stiles WB, Inui TS, et al. Physician frustration in communicating with patients. Med Care 1993;31:285–95.
25. McLafferty RB, Williams RG, Lambert AD, et al. Surgeon communication behaviors that lead patients to not recommend the surgeon to family members or friends: analysis and impact. Surgery 2006;140:616–24.
26. Eisenthal S, Koopman C, Stoeckle JD. The nature of patients' requests for physicians' help. Acad Med 1990;65:401–5.
27. Levinson W, Roter DL, Mullooly JP, et al. Physician patient communication: the relationship with malpractice claims among primary care physicians and surgeons. JAMA 1997;277:553–9.
28. Kaplan SH, Greenfield S, Ware JE. Assessing the effects of physician-patient interactions on the outcomes of chronic disease. Med Care 1989;27: S110–27.
29. Rost KM, Flavin KS, Cole K, et al. Change in metabolic control and functional status after hospitalization. Diabetes Care 1991;14:881–9.
30. Mumfor K, Schlesinger HJ, Glass GV. The effect of psychological intervention on recovery from surgery and heart attacks: an analysis of the literature. Am J Public Health 1982;72:141–51.
31. Fallowfield LJ, Hall A, Maguire GP, et al. Psychological outcomes of different treatment policies in women with early breast cancer outside a clinical trial. BMJ 1990;301:575–80.
32. Maguiro P, Pitreathly C. Key communication skills and how to acquire them. BMJ 2002;325:697700.
33. Back AL, Arnold RM, Baile WF, et al. Approaching difficult communication tasks in oncology. CA Cancer J Clin 2005;55:164–77.
34. Helft PR, Petronio S. Communication pitfalls with cancer patients: "hit-and-run" deliveries of bad news. J Am Coll Surg 2007;205:807–11.
35. Levinson W, Chaumeton N. Communication between surgeons and patients in routine office visits. Surgery 1999;125:127–34.

36. Eggly S, Penner LA, Albrecht TL, et al. Discussing bad news in the outpatient oncology clinic: rethinking current communication guidelines. J Clin Oncol 2006;24(4):716–9.
37. Sise MJ, Sise CB, Sack DI, et al. Surgeons' attitudes about communicating with patients and their families. Curr Surg 2006;63:213–8.
38. Milch RA, Dunn GP. Communication: part of the surgical armamentarium. J Am Coll Surg 2001;193:449–51.
39. Buckman R. Communication skills in palliative care: a practical guide. Neurol Clin 2001;19:989–1004.
40. Easter DW, Beach W. Competent patient care is dependent upon attending to empathetic opportunities presented during interview sessions. Curr Surg 2004; 61:313–8.
41. McCahill LE, Dunn GP, Mosenthal AC, et al. Palliation as a core surgical principle: part 2. J Am Coll Surg 2004;199(2):321–34.
42. Von Gunten CF, Ferris FD, Emanuel LL. Ensuring competency in end-of-life care: communication and relational skills. JAMA 2000;284:3051–7.
43. Traveline JM, Ruchinskas R, D'Alonzo GE. Patient-physician communication: why and how. J Am Osteopath Assoc 2005;105:13–8.
44. Klaristenfeld DD, Harrington DT, Miner TJ. Teaching palliative care and end-of-life issues: a core curriculum for surgical residents. Ann Surg Oncol 2007;14(6): 1801–6.
45. Huffman JL. Educating surgeons for the new golden hours: honing the skills of palliative care. Surg Clin North Am 2005;85(2):383–91.
46. Gordon G. Care not cure: dialogues at the transition. Patient Educ Couns 2003; 50:95–8.

# Surgical Palliative Care in Haiti

Joan L. Huffman, MD, CWS

KEYWORDS

- Palliative care • Mass casualty event • Haiti earthquake
- Wound care

> 13. We are on our scabbed backs.
>    There is the sound of whispered splashing,
>    And then this:
>    Leave them.
>                              —Patricia Smith

According to the World Health Organization, palliative care is an approach that improves the quality of life of patients and their families facing life-threatening illness through the prevention, assessment, and treatment of pain and other physical, psychosocial, and spiritual problems.[1]

The US Homeland Security definition of a catastrophic health event or mass casualty event (MCE) is "any natural or manmade incident, including terrorism, that results in a number of ill or injured persons sufficient to overwhelm the capabilities of immediate local and regional emergency and healthcare systems."[2] In summary, disaster care at its inception is a minimally acceptable care because of the diversity and volume of patients. In today's world, responders must deal not only with an austere environment with challenges to resources, access, and transport but also with physical, economic, and social difficulties made more complex by political constraints.[3]

What happens when an MCE collides with palliative care? Hurricane Katrina of 2005 is a national example. In 2010, a disaster of even greater magnitude occurred in Haiti, a Pan-American nation located just 600 miles from Florida.

## BACKGROUND

Palliative care was initially instituted for better pain control in patients with cancer. As time progressed, it expanded to include symptom control and enveloped not only the physical person but also the emotional and spiritual being. Palliative care now focuses

A version of this article was published in the 91:2 issue of Surgical Clinics of North America.
The author has nothing to disclose.
Division of Acute Care Surgery, Department of Surgery, University of Florida at Shands Jacksonville, 655 West 8th Street, 8th Floor Clinical Center, Jacksonville, FL 32209, USA
E-mail address: joan.huffman@jax.ufl.edu

Anesthesiology Clin 30 (2012) 59–71
doi:10.1016/j.anclin.2011.11.005
1932-2275/12/$ – see front matter © 2012 Elsevier Inc. All rights reserved.

on the relief of suffering, health care needs, dignity of the person, and quality of life at the end of life. It encompasses the patient's family and friends. Over the past 30 years, additional focus has been placed on the care of patients with AIDS. With the aging of the baby boomers of the North American and European populations, patients with chronic disease states (such as chronic obstructive pulmonary disease, renal failure, and decompensated coronary artery disease/congestive heart failure) are also considered now for palliative care.

What happens to palliative care when an MCE occurs? Following an MCE, there are 4 groups of patients who fall into the "not expected to survive" category: patients already under hospice/palliative care; vulnerable patients in long-term care facilities with an advanced disease (1%–2% of normal population); individuals exposed to the MCE who are expected to die; and other patients triaged due to scarce resources. Suddenly, because of an abruptly austere environment, all these patients are shifted to palliative care.

New Orleans, Louisiana, was overwhelmed with the onslaught of Hurricane Katrina. Despite the high-tech modern health care system of the United States, difficult decisions had to be made in harrowing circumstances. With generator failures, critical care equipment ceased to function, and with modern just-in-time stores and cutoff of supply lines, severe shortages of medication, food, and potable water occurred; both patients and staff suffered immensely. In these circumstances, palliative care was often the best and/or the only care that medical staff could provide. In St. Rita's Nursing Home, St. Bernard Parish, 20 miles southeast of New Orleans, staff abandoned patients whom they could not evacuate. Patricia Smith, a poet, gives voice to each of the 34 individuals who died. Particularly poignant is 13, a resident who was lucid enough to realize that they were being left to drown (see opening quote).[4]

In recognition of the events that happened post-Katrina, a recent ruling by The Joint Commission instructed that "the needs of those who may not survive catastrophic MCE and the 'existing' vulnerable populations affected by the event should be incorporated in to the planning, preparation, response and recovery management systems of all regions and jurisdictions." In addition, surge capacity should be addressed with attention to triage and rationing of supplies and personnel. A defined minimum of what is palliative care, to be made available to all, must take priority over heroic efforts toward severely injured or critically ill patients.[5] Aggressive steps have been taken to implement these recommendations in the United States; other nations are not as fortunate.

## HAITI

How does palliative care play out in even more austere circumstances? An opportunity to learn the answer arose on January 12, 2010, when a 7.0 Richter scale earthquake struck Haiti, the poorest country in the Western Hemisphere, and absolute devastation occurred. There were more than 200,000 fatalities, 300,000 injuries, and millions of displaced persons. It was a disaster of epic proportions, and even now in retrospect, one of the major TIME stories of 2010.[6,7]

## HISTORICAL PERSPECTIVE

Haitian response to the disaster and subsequent interaction with and expectations of international health care providers must be viewed based on a historical/sociocultural context, health beliefs, and the access to care. Until 1492, and contact by Christopher Columbus, the island was inhabited by indigenous peoples (Taíno/Arawak) who perished after enslavement by the Spanish. They were replaced first by the Nicaraguan slaves and soon after by Africans through the Atlantic slave trade. Eventually, compe-tition between Spanish and French interests led to the division of Hispaniola into a French western one-third and a Spanish eastern two-thirds, the modern day Haiti and Dominican Republic (DR), respectively. Haiti proved profitable to France as its richest colony for over 2 centuries.

In 1804, Haiti became the first Black republic after the slaves fought and won their independence from their colonial masters. Haiti thrived for the following century until external (exploitation by foreign investors and governments) and internal forces (polit-ical corruption, instability, and mismanagement) led to the decay of freedom, under-development, and generalized suffering. Only after the end of the Duvalier dictatorship in 1986 and the subsequent 1991 coup d'état of Jean-Bertrand Aristide (by the Toton Macoute, with US collaboration), which ended in 1994, did the most basic of infrastructures evolve under the leadership of President René Préval. This fragile system collapsed, both structurally and functionally, with the earthquake.[8]

## SOCIOCULTURAL ASPECTS

Haiti is populated by more than 9 million young individuals: 50% are younger than 20 years, and about half are rural and single. Almost everyone speaks Kreyòl (Haitian Creole), a mélange of French, African, Arawakan, Spanish, and English; however, literacy, defined as the ability to read French, is very low (rural, 20%; urban, 50%). The literacy rate is not surprising because three-quarters of the population have just a primary school education. More than 90% of all formal educational institutions are nonstate private facilities; university education is attained by only 1%.

Class hierarchy is powerful, with special focus on economic background, culture, language, and education. Hailing back to colonization, further stratification is based on skin tone. Light-skinned literate persons with access to private education maintain an elite status with most of the social, economic, and political powers, whereas dark-skinned people tend to be marginalized.[8]

The disparity is echoed in income inequality, which is one of the highest worldwide. A small elite of several thousand people includes many millionaires contrasted with the teeming slums of the capital city, Port-au-Prince (P-a-P), where the daily income may be $2. The disparity also resonates in unemployment (one-third of rural persons, one-half of metropolitan dwellers) and basic services (most rural homes have no indoor plumbing, only 10% have electricity compared with 90% with power access in metro regions). In 2008, the gross national income per capita was $653.70; more than 80% of the population lives in poverty, and 54% in abject poverty. Because of the desperate conditions, many Haitians have migrated to the United States (500,000) and Canada (Montreal, 100,000). The annual remittances of the diaspora provide $800 million of support to friends and family in the homeland. The current US recession has drasti-cally reduced remittances at a time of financial desperation in Haiti.[9,10]

An extended, elastic family unit is the basic support structure, with interdependence on clusters of units sharing a common lakou (courtyard). In more-urban nonshanty town areas, a combination of time-honored and Anglo elements existed; however, much of these elements have reverted to traditional arrangements with the explosive evolution of tent-city communities.

Fathers, often absent, hold family authority and financial responsibility, but in reality, the mothers are the poto mitan (central pillar) of the family. The most common family structure is viv avek (living with) common-law unions and their respective 5 to 7 chil-dren. Another pattern is plasaj, in which a man has more than 1 common-law wife. The man is supposed to provide for each of his wives and the children of their relationship. Legal/religious marriages are encouraged by the state and church for filial and social stability and AIDS prevention. The roles of men reside in financial provision, home maintenance, and agriculture, whereas women run the household and manage the meager budget.

At the extremes of age, elders are treated with high respect in intergenerational households, with the oldest man in the home having authority. On the other hand, children are raised with great discipline and corporal punishment. It is not uncommon for poor rural families, with hopes of better lives for their children, to give their children to foster families. Unfortunately, many of the restavèk (stay with) youths are subject to the abuses of human trafficking.[8]

## HEALTH BELIEFS

Health practices in Haiti cannot be discussed in isolation from religion and culture. Haiti has a rich religious diversity that blends Vodou (unknown percentage), Catholic (80%), and Protestant (20%) beliefs. Despite public affiliation with Christianity, most Haitians practice Vodou (the Fon word for spirit) to some degree. After Vodou was forbidden and Catholicism made mandatory, slaves gave their African gods the names of Catholic saints; this naming gave them the superficial appearance of compliance, but they were able to keep facets of their native beliefs. Other African deities are known as lwas (ancestors' spirits) and are considered guardian angels, but they may also "possess" the body of an individual, more commonly women than men. This possession can be confused with mental illness or neurologic disorders. More rural and poorer people perform Vodou rituals, but in times of crisis, even upper-class Haitians may resort to traditional faith for aid. In general, Haitians do not speak openly about Vodou.

In juxtaposition to North American/Western anthropocentric culture, that is, humans are the center of the Universe, Haitians exist in a cosmocentric culture, that is, humans are just 1 form of energy, condensed and drawn from an all-encompassing cosmic Being. The primary focus of this great Being is to bring one into harmony and synergy with the energy of the universe. The concept of the individual is that one is made up of 4 dimensions: kò kadav (body), lonbraj (shade), gwo bon-anj (big good angel), and nam/ti bon-anj (little good angel). In concert with these tenets is a hybrid model of illness and health. There should be a balance between health, the state of well-being in connectedness to nature, the nonhuman environment, family and friends, the human environment, and the invisible, the spirits, and illness, the state of being ill with or disharmony between elements of the environment. Keeping these concepts in mind, illness is thought to originate from the failure to observe rules of hygiene, ethical rules, and rules that govern how humans relate with nature. In the humoral theory, disease is caused by an imbalance of these components. Appropriate treatment is to restore equilibrium by applying treatment in the opposite direction.

Other influences are failure to observe ancestor rites and evil influence of others (human or otherwise).

Illness is classified into 3 domains: maladi Bondyè (God's disease/natural causes), treatment is by either Western medicine or doktè fey (traditional healers); maladi fè-moun mal (human magic spells); and maladi lwa or Satan (good or evil spirits), healing is by consultation with the bòkò (magician) or oungan (Vodou priest, using herbal and ritual practices, or pursuing "unnatural" causes of illness). Oungans are not adverse to biomedical treatments and may refer clients who are beyond their scope of practice. Bòkòs are professional sorcerers who can cast or undo curses/spells or, on the positive side, aid in the achievement of personal gains. Spiritual leaders, both traditional and religious, can be used as allies to encourage patients to follow medical treatments and/or to help obtain trust by serving as cotherapists. Supernatural forces are considered to be the cause of mental illness. The problem is thought to be because of a hex, curse, or failure to please the spirits of the deceased. Death is considered to be just a normal phase of the energy flow through the cycle of life, from birth to life to death to ancestor spirit.

Illness is experienced and described much differently than in Western medicine. Symptoms may be related as metaphors depending on the volatility of the circumstances, with no reference to anatomy but to energy or other natural/unnatural elements. The practitioner is expected to elicit the appropriate symptoms to make a diagnosis.[8]

## PREEARTHQUAKE ACCESS TO HEALTH CARE

The Haitian Ministère de la Santé Publique et de la Population budget for health care is $2 per person per year. About 46% of the country's medical professionals work in P-a-P, although 70% of the population lives outside P-a-P. There is high infant mortality, and the average life span of a Haitian is 61 years, with only 3.4% aged more than 65 years compared with 13% in the United States.[11,12]

There is little to no access to health care in rural areas. In the mountain village, where we provided a free clinic for 2 days on our last Haiti mission, the priest, Pere Desca, told us that his community had not seen a doctor for more than a year (Pere Desca, Fond Baptiste, Haiti, personal communication, August 2010). Sadly, more than 80% of trained doctors leave Haiti within 5 years of graduation.

Hôpital de l'Université d'État d'Haiti (HUEH) was the main clinical referral and the only 24-hour trauma center in Haiti. HUEH, known to the people of P-a-P as Hopital General, operated on an annual budget of $5 million. Hopital General, downtown near the National Palace, as well as the national medical school and nursing schools were decimated by the earthquake. An entire class of nursing students was killed. Many hospital staff were killed or injured or had to leave to care for their injured family members.

## IMMEDIATE POSTEARTHQUAKE RESPONSE BY HAITIANS

Some of the most vulnerable individuals, the residents of the collapsed Hospice Municipal, a nursing home in Delmas-2 located only a mile from the airport, were left with only the administrator and cleaner to care for them. Of the 94 residents, 6 survived the event and were left lying in the open, some on mattresses and others in the dirt, with rats picking at their overflowing diapers. A carton of water had been donated; 1 family member came with a small amount of boiled rice. Neighboring, Place de la Paix, slum people thronged to the nursing home grounds to set up tents, threatening and stealing their meager belongings. Two elderly people tried to guard the group: a blind man in a wheelchair and an old lady who brandished her walking stick. Day by day, the residents died or waited to die because of dehydration, hunger, and no medicine.[13]

Zanmi Lasante (ZL), the flagship project of Partners in Health (PIH), provided care to the multitudes that fled to Haiti's Central Plateau and Artibonite regions, set up health outposts at 4 camps for internally displaced people in P-a-P, and began working at Hopital General with the 370 remaining staff and volunteers. ZL also facilitated the placement of volunteer surgeons, physicians, and staff, as well as helped the hospital's Haitian leadership.[14]

Max Delices, the director at Hospice St Joseph (HSJ), our team's base camp, told us that before we came, he helped pull people from rubble and mobilized young volunteers to go out into the neighborhood with povidone-iodine (Betadine) and gauze to clean and dress wounds. "Everyone was a doctor in those first hours and days." He said that our visit gave hope for a future to him, the staff, and the neighborhood and that he slept for the first time in more than a week (Max Delices, HSJ, P-a-P, Haiti, personal communication, January 2010).

## EARLY RELIEF MISSION RESPONSE

Nearly 1000 members of the American College of Surgeons responded to the disaster. Some of the earliest surgical help arrived from Miami on January 13th, and triage began under tents at the United Nations compound just outside P-a-P. Initial care included intravenous (IV) hydration, morphine analgesia, and oral antibiotics. Amputations were done under local anesthesia. Tetanus toxoid arrived 24 hours later, and the team began to operate in conjunction with an Israeli team. Over the next week, a Civil War camp of tents, additional supplies, and specialists evolved.[15]

The principle of justice was used as disaster teams focused on potentially survivable yet severely injured earthquake survivors. A Haitian facility agreed to provide palliative care to individuals who were under coma, in vegetative states, or minimally responsive or whose families opted for comfort care only. Staff of this facility were trained on the US Naval Ship (USNS) COMFORT for 3 days; supplies were also provided.[16]

A. Brent Eastman, MD, FACS, responded to a hospital 1 mile from the earthquake epicenter, where he scrubbed under a broken faucet and operated on a patient with upper extremity compartment syndrome, with no electric cautery, ketamine-only anesthesia, and no monitoring. The patient's arm was saved, and the patient was satisfied with the care provided. The American team learned the necessity of sensitivity to working in another culture and quickly learned to invite the Haitian technicians to scrub with them and to give the Haitian doctors first choice of operating "rooms" and anesthesiologists. Dr Eastman said, "We were there to help, not to dominate and occupy."[17]

Other important lessons learned were the necessity of reliance on basic physical diagnostic skills, with no laboratories, radiographs, or computed tomographic scans. The doctors had "to look at the patient, talk to the patient and touch the patient," said Sylvia Campbell, MD, FACS. In such dire circumstances, it was a pleasure for physicians and a comfort to patients to participate in the laying on of hands.

A surgical resident, Joseph Sakran, MD, learned the lesson of his young career as he watched a teenage patient with late-stage tetanus and horrific spasmodic contractions. The only care available was supportive. The patient was moved to a dark, quiet room, both for his comfort as he lay dying and to take him out of the tent where his situation had terrified the other patients.[15]

The severity, complexity, and number of survivors taxed the limits of the USNS COMFORT, which arrived within 8 days of the disaster. In a staff meeting, colleagues discussed the difficult decisions confronting them, such as ventilator capacity, blood product use, the conflict between routine trauma management and disaster management, and the allotment of scarce resources. One option included setting up palliative care facilities at triage sites onshore, but a surgeon nixed the idea because he was aghast at the concept of having a tent of dying patients adjacent to a medevac site, and he found it unpalatable to give a bed to a moribund patient. However, nursing argued that a bed out of the sun and painkillers were more humane than leaving the individual to "die in the street under the sun like a dog." During the brief meeting, 2 patients died, 1 in the operating room.[16]

Two doctors, in the Fundamental Disaster Management (FDM) subcommittee of the Society of Critical Care Medicine (SCCM), described their situations on arriving at P-a-P. One was Dennis Amundson, DO, FCCM, who led an 18-member intensivist team of respiratory therapists and nurses as the initial staff on the USNS COMFORT. They cared for critically ill patients in a 40-bed intensive care unit (ICU) at full capacity for 3 weeks. They had to make difficult triage decisions, focusing their attention on patients who "weren't necessarily the sickest, but had the best opportunity for long term survival." Other patients were kept as comfortable as possible until their demise.

The other doctor, James Geiling, MD, FCCM, and 8 nurses from Dartmouth Medical Center teamed up with PIH at Hopital General to set up a postoperative/ICU tent adjacent to an improvised operating room in one of the remaining single- or double-story buildings; all multistory buildings had collapsed, "it looked like it had been bombed."[18] Their team provided critical care to crush and gunshot wound survivors with only a small supply of antibiotics, an oxygen tank, and a blood pressure cuff (until the cuff was stolen). Dr Geiling said, "My ICU management was how strong was their pulse, how pale was their tongue and how fast they were breathing." It was ICU care in name only; in fact, it was wound care and physical diagnosis.[19] As more assistance arrived, teams from the United States and around the world pooled and collaborated. Medical providers worked around the clock in the first hours and days, with more than half of the team members requiring IV hydration; after a few days, operations were cut back to daylight hours only to allow conservation of provider energy because it quickly became obvious that the number was not going to decrease anytime in the foreseeable future.[18]

The earthquake occurred while the 39th Critical Care Congress, SCCM, was in session in Miami, Florida; at that very time, discussions were underway to initiate Fundamental Critical Care Support (FCCS) training in the DR. How ironic because Haiti was not the only country affected by the earthquake disaster, as survivors rushed to the DR, where 75% of the 7.5 million residents use the public hospital system. An SCCM Disaster Field Team (DFT) was quickly formed, and it did an initial assessment of the overflowing Jimani, DR, clinic at the Haiti-DR border and the 70 public ICU beds in the entire DR, which were staffed with nurses with minimal critical care education, had no respiratory therapists, and had minimal equipment. In 3 days, the DFT set up and subsequently taught the earthquake disaster portions of both FDM and Pediatric FCCS to 60 medical residents and nurses, who immediately went to work at the Jimani clinic; 3 weeks later, a repeat course educated another 30 staff members, and a new 6-bed ICU was set up in Barahona, DR. The health systems of both countries of Hispaniola will remain stressed for an extended period.[20]

A team from Operation Smile provided palliative care for a 4-year-old child with more than 85% flame burns, who was not able to access care until postinjury day 3. The best care they could provide was to remove the child's burnt clothing in the operating room, with only morphine for analgesia and silver sulfadiazine (Silvadene) and soft gauze to cover the wounds. The USNS COMFORT was unable to provide burn care, and there were no other burn facilities available. The child's mother was gently told the bad news, and the child was kept as comfortable as possible until his immediate demise.[21]

## PERSONAL EXPERIENCE

I had the opportunity to respond to the earthquake disaster 1 week after the event. Our host was the HSJ, not a hospice in American terms but a guesthouse for visiting health care providers and a refuge for people from the countryside, who came to P-a-P seeking medical care. In addition, there was a maternal-infant clinic on-site, and educational scholarships were administered.[22] The building and its surrounding walls had pancaked down as so many did in the few fatal seconds; however, there were no injuries on-site, although one of the directors rode the building down. The staff secured the premises with corrugated aluminum barriers and salvaged mattresses and cooking implements from the rubble. Due to limited space within the confines of our walls, we multi purposed the area: during the day, we held an on-site clinic, at night the same location served as our living room, dining room and bedroom. We slept on the ground with the staff and shared a meal of beans and rice each evening.

Our base was in the Christ Roi neighborhood, a "Red Zone" and a poor area that the government did not prioritize for care. The Disaster Medical Assistance Team (DMAT), shown on the international news, was at the Hopital General in downtown P-a-P and in other "Green Zones" such as Pètionville. Our 13-member team consisted of a surgeon; a family practice intern; a trauma psychologist; a medical nurse practitioner; 2 physician assistants, 1 medical and the other surgical; 2 registered nurses; a social worker; a public health specialist; an anthropologist; and 2 unarmed security men. Among them, 5 members were fluent in *Kreyòl*. We partnered with 12 local paramedical volunteers to treat people with little to no access to health care in the local neighborhood, the Acra district tent city several blocks away, and the huge Solino tent city set up on a soccer field in one of the city's slum areas.

Our 20 crates of medical supplies were either lost or subverted, so we were limited to the contents of 13 duffel bags that we hand-carried on the chartered flight from Miami. Our supplies consisted of basic wound/fracture care materials, IV/oral rehydration solutions, and basic adult and pediatric medications. These minimal resources were expanded with some additional pediatric drugs salvaged from the HSJ clinic and donated by the Catholic Relief Services and the International Medical Corps.

In 5 days, we treated more than 1000 people from our seemingly bottomless duffel bags; it was truly an example of what can be done with a few supplies and a lot of imagination, a modern day feeding of the multitudes with 7 loaves and 7 fishes. A small contingent of the team held daily clinics at HSJ, but the remainder worked in *Klinik Mobil* (mobile clinics) in the tent cities. We enlisted local men to construct temporary shaded or screened patient areas; doors balanced on chairs served as examination tables.

We did not see any actively dying people, but the mangled arm of a motorcyclist protruded from the debris in the street. Near Hopital General, body after body was carried into an overflowing morgue. Women crouched curbside, cooking with charcoal, while human excrement ran by their feet; the overpowering sweet stench of death permeated the air, intermingled with the acrid smoke of burning bodies and garbage.

Of the disease categories, 50% were surgical and 50% medical. Every person we examined had lost either a family member or a friend; some had lost all. Many had witnessed the deaths, the tragedy just an arm's length away, yet unreachable. We dealt with the after effects, both physical and emotional. No matter what the presenting problem was, everyone complained of *tet fe mal, vant doule*, and *verti* (headache, stomach pain, and dizziness). The source of their ailments was not only acute injury but also ongoing austere conditions, dehydration, hunger, and enormous stress. Neither the patients nor their accompanying person was turned away empty-handed, everyone was given a packet of over-the-counter pain relief and antacids as a simple palliative measure.

Five patients required transport by private vehicle to Hopital General: a man with severe head injury, who was carried into the *Klinik* with seizures and a distended tender abdomen; a woman with cauda equina syndrome; a man with a lumbar fracture, who was brought on a blanket into the *Klinik* (I made him a thoracolumbar brace from a cardboard box and 2 Ace bandages); and 2 infants with refractory dehydration.

We did not have the capability to provide any extensive operative interventions, except for wound debridement and digital amputations. All surgical procedures were done under local or regional anesthesia, supplemented by oral ibuprofen and emotional support by the team's psychologist or social worker. One young girl passed out as I extracted a chunk of concrete from her infected ankle. We worked side by side with young paramedical volunteers. Wound after wound was cleansed, debrided, and dressed. Crushed and fractured limbs were assessed by palpation and functional status. Those fractured limbs that were ambulatory were treated with Ace wraps, and those that were not were reduced as close to an anatomic position as possible and splinted; the fractures were more than a week old, and Hopital General was only dealing with open devastating wounds and fractures.

A woman presented with an upper extremity crush injury. I am certain that she must have had compartment syndrome early on, but her limb and life were saved because the skin and tissues of her forearm split open. I amputated 3 digits and widely debrided necrotic tissue from her hand. As I operated, in a church courtyard, surrounded by curious children and an anxious sister, doing a case that in the United States would have been done under general anesthesia, she laid still and stoic without even a whimper. After the wound was dressed and a sling was applied, she thanked us effusively for a handful of ibuprofen, the first pain medicine she had received after 9 days of horrible pain. She returned to our host clinic for follow-up. The stumps were healing nicely, and the swelling in her hand was markedly reduced. Unfortunately, en route to the clinic she was caught in a motorcycle accident and sustained deep abrasions to her legs. We treated those wounds as well.

There were many dehydrated babies. Most of them were treated with oral rehydration and a few with IV rehydration. One baby was so badly dehydrated that we could not obtain IV access and had to revert to an old technique called hypodermoclysis, a subcutaneous infusion of fluids.

Two desperate parents brought their only surviving daughter to the *Klinik*; they had seen the crushing death of her 2 siblings. The girl was hyperventilating and had not slept since the event, so had the parents. We administered diphenhydramine for sedation and worked to calm her. We counseled her parents and taught the whole family breathing and relaxation exercises.

At our first Solino *Klinik*, a grandmother invited us into her sparse bedsheet tent to proudly show off her daughter's newborn infant. On our last day, I saw the grandmother gently plaiting her daughter's hair, and I inquired about the baby, "*Tibebé a mouri...*" The young mother, too dehydrated and malnourished, was unable to breast-feed. I did not know enough *Kreyòl* to properly give my condolences, but I sat for a few moments and shared their silence.

## THREE MONTHS POSTEARTHQUAKE

A team of 6 members returned to Christ Roi in April 2010. It was a joyous reunion for returning team members, staff, and neighborhood acquaintances. HSJ was again our base. The building was being demolished by hand; men were working with pickaxes, crowbars, and sledgehammers. A temporary clinic with 2 examination rooms and a pharmacy was functioning 3 days a week on-site, and half-day school sessions, AM and PM, were being held, with all children receiving a hot lunch. A dormitory constructed of corrugated aluminum, with twin beds and fans, was now our home; flush toilets (with a bucket) and a shower (bucket bath) stall our amenities.

On this visit, we primarily assisted the Haitian primary care physicians and pediatricians in the HSJ clinic and also held clinics on their days off. We held one *Klinik Mobil* at a tent city in Pegueyville, outside Pètionville, at the request of 2 Brooklyn aid workers who had discovered a band of orphaned boys dropped off and abandoned at the site. We treated their wounds and worms and also saw the many women and children who queued for treatment. Our presence was announced by *radio bouch* (word of mouth), and so a motorcyclist dropped off a man with a freshly broken femur. We made him as comfortable as possible by laying him in the shade, reducing his limb, and giving him ibuprofen. Our transport van had gone on other errands, so it was not available. Shortly thereafter, a van with missionaries arrived, and we asked them to take the man to the hospital, but "it was out of their way." The missionaries took all the orphans, except for a boy with an open cleft palate and extremity deformities because he would be too much trouble. Abandoned again, now without his "wolf pack" for protection and aid, the child will surely die. At the end of the day, once our van returned, we transported the injured man to the hospital. The preoperative and postoperative tents of the DMAT were gone, but a good number of aid workers and tents remained, and in a more organized fashion. We expedited the injured man and his wife through the admission process, but the facility was reluctant to provide treatment.

We saw more than 500 patients on this trip; only 12% had surgical complaints, three-quarters had wounds and abscesses, and the remainder had hernias, congenital anomalies, and tumors. We treated the acute issues and referred the others to the Hopital; they probably will not be seen. The triune complaint of headache, stomach pain, and dizziness was pervasive. Most people were eating only 1 or 2 meager meals a day. New complaints of back pain echoed. At daytime, they were laboring to demolish or repair their homes, and at night, they were sleeping on the ground, some now with real tents. We could not provide food or better shelter, so we gave them over-the-counter pain relief and antacids; we added vitamins for everyone, young and old. Amazingly, despite malnutrition, dehydration, and gross contamination, wounds were healing well.

## SIX MONTHS POSTEARTHQUAKE

We continue to learn from our experiences and have made more contacts. On this trip, we were able to acquire prescription medications for general medical and infective conditions. We also received many donations of a wider variety of over-the-counter medications. Although our treatments still remained largely symptomatic and palliative, we were able to advance to providing more focused medical care.

On a third trip to Haiti, we spent 1 day assisting in the HSJ clinic, which had now expanded to include a laboratory facility, an enlarged pharmacy, and a large sturdy tent with a triage area and 2 examination rooms. Because we had the perspective of time, the circumstances, and some familiarity with the staff, our role was not only to provide medical/surgical care but also to observe the *Klinik* system and make recommendations for improvements. We met with the visiting board members to discuss our suggestions. We also held *Klinik Mobil*, returning to the Acra neighborhood for 2 days, which was set up in a church just outside Cite Soleil (a notoriously dangerous slum) for 1 day. Clean water seemed to be readily available in P-a-P; however, the air was heavy with particulate matter, and there was an increase in respiratory and eye irritation complaints.

A mother brought her 2 desperately ill infants, both in acute respiratory distress with high fever. We initiated treatment with oral infant acetaminophen and antibiotics. We did not have a nebulizer, so we used metered dose inhaler treatments instead. Because of the severity of their illness, we transported them to Hopital General but were turned away because the ward was full of actively dying children. Our physician assistant dedicated hours to treating these children, with small doses of adult prednisone and oral rehydration. By the end of the day, they were much improved, but we had to leave; we have hope for the children but no knowledge of their outcome.

On this trip, we were invited to journey to a secluded mountain village, Fond Baptiste, perched high above the plain of Artibonite. Our trip took more than 4 hours, with half of the team balanced precariously atop supplies at the back of a 4-wheel drive pickup truck, vying with mules, goats, and pedestrians for the road. Health care was a distant memory to those people; however, the air was cool and clean but the water not as much. Extensive dental caries and worm infestations were common. We saw more elderly patients, most in surprisingly good health. But many untreated surgical conditions were observed in patients of all ages, especially hernias.

Our visit had been timed to coincide with the weekly market to maximize the number of patients we could see in a 2-day visit. By chance, after a walk through the market at the end of clinic hours, we came upon a woman with a large arm tumor, and she was sitting on her porch rocking in pain. On physical examination, the mass was 20 × 20 cm, firmly fixed to her upper humerus, and exquisitely tender on palpation. We gave her the only narcotics we had, from the private script of a team member, and invited her daughter to bring her to the clinic the next day. In the morning, she came for a formal visit. She had received a little relief from our medication but had slept a little, the first rest in quite awhile. We gave her all the remaining methocarbamol and ibuprofen from our pharmacy. We have been trying to make arrangements between our contacts in HSJ, Fond Baptiste, and a team of orthopedic physicians who provide service at Hospital Sacre Coeur in Milot near Cap Haïtien. Unfortunately, because of the plethora of intervening events in Haiti over the past 3 months, we have not been able to set up for her either a scheduled appointment or a travel to the distant site over harrowing roads; by the time we can make arrangements, it surely will be too late to be of benefit. If we are able to return to that location and she still lives, we will be certain to take some more potent medication especially for her.[23]

## SUMMARY

Sometimes, our missions are like a series of throwing 1 starfish at a time into the vast ocean, an immeasurable task, but it is worth it all to the few starfish that are returned to their briny home. Despite their dire circumstances, our Haitian patients attend the *Klinik* looking their best, shoes polished, little girls' hair neatly braided, and young boys spiffed and polished. They are polite, enormously grateful for the simplest of examinations, and pleasantly surprised by our gift of vitamins to one and all. Perhaps, the greatest palliative care we provide is the assurance that there are still caring individuals in the world and the hope for a better tomorrow.

Palliative care is implemented in an individually designed fashion; disaster care is organized to provide the best for the most in austere circumstances. When these 2 elements struck head-on in a little known yet very locally accessible nation, with only a very basic infrastructure before the disaster, a challenging situation occurred. Preparation and planning on the part of those planning to deploy must include all aspects of emergency response, including palliative care. Yet, despite the proximity of Haiti, there had been little general education in the United States about the background of our sister nation; understanding the history and culture of a locale is essential to provide sensitive, appropriate care that will be accepted by the local population. Early wound and fracture intervention was key not only to help prevent progression to limb loss, sepsis, and death but also to increase mobility, a crucial necessity for homeless survivors who daily had to seek food and water.

When surgeons respond to a disaster situation, they will encounter suffering on an enormous scale. Although active triage and treatment are undertaken, in some instances, proper intervention is not an operation or primary disease control but to give comfort and restore hope. Palliative care can mean giving a man a stick to bite on while his leg is amputated, touching the shoulder of a mother whose child was buried under the collapse of the school building, or bringing a smile to the face of a child who has not smiled for 6 months.

## EXTENDED CHALLENGES

As if all the past political and socioeconomic factors compounded by the tragic earthquake are not enough for the Haitian people to bear, hurricane force winds and rain, a cholera epidemic, and incendiary violence caused by an uncertain presidential election may further test Haiti's health care availability and function, as well as the ability for foreign nongovernmental organizations to safely be able to continue to gain access to the country and give ongoing care. For most Haitians, the experience of daily living is an exercise in palliative care. But they persevere saying, "beyond mountains there are more mountains," a common Haitian proverb that the natives live by—despite all the challenges they have had to overcome, there are yet more challenges to come, and still, they hope for a better future.

## ACKNOWLEDGMENTS

The author wishes to acknowledge all the care providers who responded to Haiti in the hour of need and those who continue to respond. To give full credit to all the team members and volunteers who worked side by side with the author, please see the Men Anpil Web site (www.men-anpil.org).[24]

## REFERENCES

1. WHO definition of palliative care. World Health Organization. 2010. Available at:http://www.who.int/cancer/palliative/definition/en/. Accessed December 19, 2010.
2. The White House. Homeland Security Presidential Directives/HSPD-21. Definition of catastrophic health event (i.e. mass casualty event). October 18, 2007. Available at: http://ncdmph.usuhs.edu/documents/hspd-21.pdf. Accessed December 19, 2010.
3. Briggs SM. The role of civilian surgical teams in response to international disasters. Bull Am Coll Surg 2010;95(1):13–7.
4. Smith P. 34. Blood dazzler. Minneapolis (MN): Coffee House Press; 2008.
5. Bogucki S, Jubanyik K. Triage, rationing and palliative care in disaster planning. Biosecur Bioterror 2009;7(2):221–4.
6. Elliot M. Haiti's agony. TIME Special Report: Haiti's tragedy. January 25, 2010. p. 30–6.
7. Clinton B. What Haiti needs. TIME Special Report: Haiti's tragedy. January 25, 2010. p. 37.

8. WHO/PAHO. Culture and mental health in Haiti: a literature review. Geneva (Switzerland): WHO; 2010.

9. World Statistics Pocketbook/United Nations Statistics Division. Last update in UN data: 14 May 2010. Available at: http://data.un.org/CountryProfile.aspx?crName= Haiti (GNI data). Accessed January 7, 2011.

10. Central Intelligence Agency. The world factbook (The on-line factbook is updated weekly) (poverty data). Available at: https://www.cia.gov/library/ publications/the-world-factbook/geos/ha.html#top. Accessed December 19, 2010.

11. Responding to the Emergency at L'Hôpital Université d'État d'Haïti: a first step in-rebuilding Haiti's public health care system. In: Proceedings of Friends of L'Hôpital Université d'État d'Haïti in conjunction with Partners in Health. March 31, 2010.

12. Ramnarace C. The forgotten victims: Haiti's elderly. AARP Bulletin. Available at: http://www.cynthiaramnarace.com/yahoo_site_admin/assets/docs/Help_for_Haiti_ Earthquakes_0610.192115005.pdf. Accessed February 13, 2011.

13. de Montesquiou A. Elderly at Haiti hospice going without aid, waiting to die. Available at: http://www.huffingtonpost.com/2010/001/17/elderly-at-hospice_n_ 426324.html?view=screen. Accessed January 17, 2010.

14. Partners in health earthquake response. Available at: http://www.standwithhaiti. org. Accessed December 19, 2010.

15. Schneidman DS. Surgeons respond to the needs of a broken nation. Bull Am Coll Surg 2010;95(6):6–9, 12–20.

16. Etienne M, Powell C, Faux B. Disaster relief in Haiti: a perspective from the neurologists on the USNS COMFORT. 2010. Available at: http://www.thelancet.com/ neurology. Accessed December 19, 2010.

17. Eastman AB. Haiti impressions. Bull Am Coll Surg 2010;95(6):9–11.

18. Ben-Achour S. Casualties and limits confront Navy Hospital Ship. Shots – NPR's Health Blog. Available at: http://www.npr.org/blogs/health/2010/01/casualties_ and_limits_strike_h.html. Accessed January 24, 2010.

19. Kilgore C. Work in Haiti leaves mark on volunteers. American College of Surgeons. Surgery News March 2010;6(3):1, 4.

20. SCCM members provide relief to disaster victims. Critical Connections. SCCM 2010;9(2):1–117.

21. Critical care at a critical time. Critical Connections. SCCM 2010;9(2):8–9.

22. Oelkers N. Blog from the field: Haiti February 6–19. Operation Smile blog. Available at: http://www.operationsmile.org/haiti/haiti-week-2.html. Accessed February 14, 2010.

23. Hospice Saint Joseph. Available at: http://www.hospicesaintjoseph.org. Accessed December 19, 2010.

24. Author's Medical Mission Web site. Men Anpil (Many Hands). Available at: http:// www.men-anpil.org. Accessed December 19, 2010.

# SECTION 2:
# Pain Management

Edited by Sugantha Ganapathy, MBBS and Vincent Chan, MD

# Paravertebral Blocks

Jacques E. Chelly, MD, PhD, MBA

KEYWORDS

• Paravertebral block • Epidural • Pain • Ultrasound

Epidural analgesia is still considered the gold standard for postoperative pain relief after many thoracoabdominal surgeries. In many patients, comorbidities and patient factors preclude the use of epidural analgesia, such as coagulopathy. Intravenous narcotics relieve pain at rest reasonably but fail to provide an acceptable level of pain relief with activities such as coughing and walking. Thus, there is a need for alternate analgesic techniques for this group of patients. Some new techniques have been described, such as the transversus abdominis plane block, and some older techniques have been rejuvenated, such as the paravertebral blocks.

Paravertebral blocks were initially described in the early twentieth century. Their use was reintroduced in1979 by Eason and Wyatt.[1,2] However, it is really over the past 15 years that paravertebral block has generated significant interest initially for the management of patients undergoing breast surgery and inguinal hernia repair. Today, evidence supports the concept that they are as effective as epidural blocks for perioperative pain management without many of the side effects of neuraxial techniques (Table 1).

The use of paravertebral block has been shown in a retrospective analysis to delay the recurrence of tumors and the development of metastases.[3] These data are consistent with those demonstrating that the use of regional anesthesia (especially epidural) has similar effects on patients undergoing prostate cancer resection. The possible mechanisms involved not only the prevention of the stress response by the regional technique but also the possibility that the beneficial effects are the result of the associated opioid-sparing effects. Thus opioids have been shown to stimulate growth factors and diminish immunologic response.

## PARAVERTEBRAL ANATOMY

The paravertebral space extends from the cervical spine to the sacrum.[4–8] At each level, especially at the thoracic level, it is a space of triangular shape limited anteriorly by the parietal pleura, medially by the posterolateral aspect of the vertebra and the intervertebral foramen, laterally by the parietal pleura, and posteriorly by the

Division of Acute Interventional Perioperative Pain and Regional Anesthesia, Department of Anesthesiology, University of Pittsburgh Medical Center, Posner Pain Center, Presbyterian Shadyside Hospital, Aiken Medical Building, 532 South Aiken Avenue, Suite 407, Pittsburgh, PA 15232, USA
E-mail address: chelje@anes.upmc.edu

Anesthesiology Clin 30 (2012) 75–90
doi:10.1016/j.anclin.2011.12.001
1932-2275/12/$ – see front matter © 2012 Elsevier Inc. All rights reserved.

**Table 1**
**Comparison of epidural with continuous paravertebral block**

|  | Epidural | Continuous Paravertebral Block |
|---|---|---|
| Laterality | Bilateral | As needed |
| Hypotension | Frequent | Infrequent |
| Postoperative Nausea and Vomiting | Frequent | No |
| Urinary Retention | Frequent | No |
| Pruritus | Frequent | No |
| Risk of Spinal Cord Injury | Low | Extremely Low |
| Risk of Respiratory Depression | Yes | No |
| Preservation of Forced Vital Capacity After Thoracotomy | 55% of preoperative | 75% of preoperative |
| Degree of Neural Blockade | Partial (SEPs maintained) | Complete (SEPs ablated) |
| Motor Blockade Outside Surgical Dermatomes | Yes | Minimal |
| Severity of Bleeding Complications | High | Moderate |
| Thromboprophylaxis | Complicated | Simple |

*Abbreviation:* SEP, somatosensory evoked potential.
*Data from* Refs.[79–84]

costotransverse ligament (**Figs. 1** and **2**). The depth of the paravertebral space has been demonstrated to vary according to the level: more superficial at the cervical level and deeper at the lumbar level. Between T4 and T8, the depth of the paravertebral space is also dependent on body mass index, age, and gender and is more difficult to predict. In contrast, between T9 and T12, the depth of the paravertebral space is more predictable and mostly depends on the level at which the block is performed.

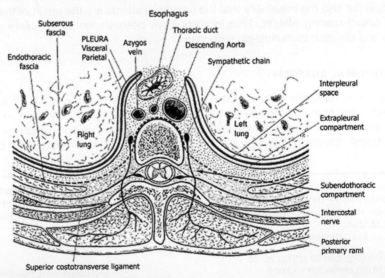

**Fig. 1.** Anatomy of the paravertebral space.

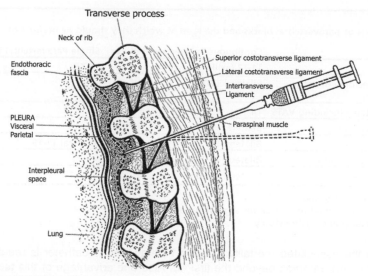

Fig. 2. Needle positioning.

## INDICATIONS

For anesthesia,[9] the indications are limited to mostly breast surgery,[10–15] inguinal hernia repair,[16–18] lithotripsy,[19] and video-assisted thoracic surgery (VATS). For breast surgery, paravertebral blocks are performed at the level of T1 to T6, especially when the surgery is associated with an axillary dissection.[20] For inguinal hernia repair, single blocks are performed at the level of T10 to L2.

The most frequent indication for paravertebral blocks is perioperative management of pain.[21–25] For surgeries associated with mild to moderate pain, such as limited inguinal hernia repair and minimally invasive cardiac surgery, single-injection paravertebral blocks are used.[26–29] For minor abdominal surgery, such as laparoscopic cholecystectomy; radical prostatectomy[30]; and hysterectomy, bilateral single paravertebral blocks are used. For major surgery, such as those associated with the placement of a chest tube[31–33]; major abdominal surgery (colon resection, debulking, pancreatectomy, liver resection)[34–37]; cardiac procedures; pelvic surgery (cystectomy, hysterectomy with node dissection); urologic procedures such as partial or complete nephrectomy; and open or laparoscopic surgery with a midline approach, a bilateral continuous paravertebral approach is recommended. In the case of a VATS[38–41] or an open thoracotomy[42–49] and a partial or complete nephrectomy, using a lateral approach and unilateral placement of a paravertebral catheter may be adequate. In this regard, it is important to recognize that most postoperative pain results from the surgical trauma and not from the skin incision. Therefore, even in the case of a laparoscopic approach, the use of a continuous paravertebral block is indicated. This point was recently illustrated by the limited benefits produced by the use of single paravertebral blocks in patients undergoing VATS. The level at which the paravertebral catheter is placed is presented in **Table 2**.

Continuous paravertebral block has also been effective in the management of pain in patients with multiple rib fractures.[50–52] In this indication, they have also been demonstrated to improve pulmonary function, reduce the need for intubation, and

**Table 2**
**Indications of paravertebral blocks and the level at which they should be performed**

|  | Continuous Paravertebral Blocks | Single Paravertebral Blocks |
|---|---|---|
| Breast | T1-T2 (axillary dissection) | T2-T6 |
| Esophagectomy/Bariatric Surgery | Bilateral T2-T3 | — |
| Thoracotomy Including VATS | T4-T5 | — |
| Liver Resection | Bilateral T6-T7 | — |
| Umbilical Hernia | Bilateral T8 | Bilateral T7-T9 |
| Abdominal Surgery | Bilateral T8-T9 | — |
| Pelvic Surgery[a,b] | Bilateral T11-T12 | T10-L1[c] |

[a] Including rectal surgery.
[b] Not a recommended technique for vaginal hysterectomy.
[c] Prostatectomy and hysterectomy.

decrease the associated mortality. Usually 1 paravertebral catheter is required for every 3 to 4 rib fractures beyond the first rib. Also one advantage of this technique is that it can be used in patients who receive enoxaparin for thromboprophylaxis. Thromboprophylaxis with enoxaparin is a contradiction for epidural.

Paravertebral blocks are also indicated for acute and chronic pain[10,53–62] and labor.[63–65]

## TECHNIQUES
### Classic Approach

Over time, several techniques have been described that can be differentiated into either blind or ultrasound guided.

Irrespective of the technique and before the block is performed, the patient is properly positioned, in most cases in the sitting position, but, occasionally and especially in trauma patients, these blocks are performed in the lateral position. These blocks should be performed in an area with full monitoring and readily available resuscitation equipment. Baseline vital signs are obtained to ensure that the patient is stable hemodynamically. A combination of midazolam and fentanyl is titrated depending on the patient's age; weight; prior history of pain and opioid use, anxiolytics, and alcohol; and hemodynamic stability. However, it should be recognized that with a carefully performed local anesthesia, it is possible to perform these blocks without any need for sedation. In elderly and very elderly patients in whom sedation is indicated, 0.5 mg of midazolam and 25 µg of fentanyl are often adequate. In young and healthy patients, 1 mg of midazolam and 50 µg of fentanyl is often used. This can be repeated according to the needs and condition of the patient. In most cases, no more than 2 mg of midazolam and 100 µg of fentanyl are required.

There are basically 3 ways to establish the level at which these blocks are performed:

1. C7
2. The lower border of the scapula (T7-T80)
3. The iliac crest (L4-L5).

Sometimes it is recommended to use 2 of these landmarks to confirm the exact level.

## BLIND TECHNIQUES
### Classic Approach

Originally, the identification of the paravertebral space was dependent on advancing the needle 1 to 2 cm after contacting the posterior surface of the transverse process. This is a technique we have used very successfully limiting our advancement to no more than 1 cm beyond the transverse process. Basically in this case, the superior border of the spinous process is identified. The site of introduction of the needle is 2.5 cm lateral from the spinous process. Before performing the block, the area is disinfected with chlorhexidine, and lidocaine 1% is injected locally using a 3.75-cm 25-gauge safety needle (B-Braun, Bethlehem, PA, USA). For single paravertebral block, a 22-gauge Tuohy needle (B-Braun, Bethlehem, PA, USA) is introduced perpendicularly to contact the posterior surface of the transverse process. When the transverse process is contacted, the distance between the skin and the transverse process is established; the needle is then withdrawn to the skin and reintroduced 1 cm beyond the transverse process at a 15° to 60° angle, allowing the positioning of the needle below the transverse process (**Fig. 3**). It is possible to experience a loss of resistance when the needle is pushed beyond the transverse process through the costotransverse ligament. If the block is performed in the upper thoracic level, the angle necessary to position the needle in the paravertebral space may have to be increased. If bone contact is established during the positioning of the needle, the needle should be withdrawn to the skin and reoriented using a greater angle. While placing a paravertebral catheter, it is not unusual that the location of the transverse process is established using a 25-gauge spinal needle (finder needle). This is followed by the placement of an 18-gauge Tuohy introducing needle in the paravertebral space.

Once the needle is positioned in the desired paravertebral space, 5 mL of either 1.0% (anesthesia) or 0.5% (analgesia) ropivacaine is slowly injected after negative aspiration for blood. If blood is aspirated, the needle is withdrawn and repositioned. When an introducer 18-gauge Tuohy needle is used, before injecting any local anesthetics in the paravertebral space, a drop technique can be used to verify that the tip of the needle is not intrapleural or in the lung. This is achieved by placing a drop of ropivacaine on the top of the needle, and the patient is asked to breathe deeply. If the ropivacaine drop follows the breathing pattern, this is considered as positive and the needle is repositioned. If the ropivacaine drop is not affected by the breathing pattern, it is considered that the needle is not intrathoracic. In this case, the needle is

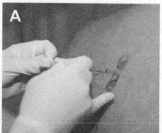 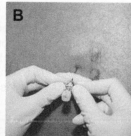 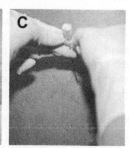

**Fig. 3.** Performance of a paravertebral block. (*A*) Introduction of the needle perpendicular to the skin in search of the transverse process. (*B*) After contacting the transverse process, the needle is pulled to the skin and the fingers are placed 1 cm beyond the depth of the transverse process. (*C*) The needle is introduced at a 45° angle to be place in the paravertebral space below the transverse process.

connected to the tubing allowing the slow injection of 5 mL of 1.0% or 0.5% ropivacaine using a 10-mL syringe. If an introducer 18-gauge Tuohy needle is used and the needle is well positioned, the injection of ropivacaine should be easy (does not offer a lot of resistance). If the injection of ropivacaine offers resistance, the 18-gauge needle is withdrawn and repositioned. After the injection is completed, either the process is repeated at another level in the case of a single paravertebral block or the paravertebral 22-gauge catheter (B-Braun, Bethlehem, PA, USA) is introduced in the paravertebral space in the case of a continuous paravertebral block. Usually, the introduction of the catheter is easy. However, there are times, despite the injection of ropivacaine being easy, when it is not possible to push the catheter beyond the tip of the needle. In this case, the catheter is first withdrawn and then the needle is rotated 180° to reposition the bevel in the opposite direction. After the rotation of the needle is complete, the catheter is reintroduced. If despite this maneuver the catheter cannot be easily introduced, the introducing needle is withdrawn and repositioned and everything is repeated as previously described. The paravertebral catheter is usually positioned 3 to 4 cm beyond the tip of the needle. After the introducing Tuohy needle is withdrawn and the catheter is secured in place using benzoin and Steri-Strips (3M St. Paul, MN, USA), an additional 10 mL of 0.5% ropivacaine is slowly injected verifying negative aspiration for blood at least every 5 mL. If blood is aspirated, the injection is stopped and the catheter is repositioned.

The administration of 10 mL of local anesthetic leads to a spread of $3.5 \pm 1.5$ dermatomal segments. Although in more than 70% the spread occurs in the paravertebral space, in 10% a "cloud" distribution occurs and in 7% there is an intercostal spread (**Fig. 4**). The type of spread is not predictable by the quality of the block. Irrespective of the distribution, it is estimated that paravertebral block fails in 6% of patients. This success rate is much higher than that of thoracic epidural.

### Loss-of-Resistance Techniques

It is possible to localize the paravertebral space using the same loss-of-resistance technique as the one used to identify the epidural space. This can only be achieved when using an 18- or a lower-gauge Tuohy needle. In this case, a couple of options are available.

### Classic technique

It is the same approach that is used to identify the epidural space. A Tuohy needle mounted to a loss-of-resistance syringe filled with saline is advanced until resistance is lost.

### Pressure transducer approach

The 18-gauge Tuohy needle is connected to a pressure transducer via pressure tubing.[66] When the needle penetrates the paravertebral space, the pressure registered by the transducer suddenly decreases. If the needle is introduced too far, it is possible to reach the pleura and/or epidural space. This technique does not allow to distinguish among the 3 possible locations unless the needle is carefully advanced.

### Neurostimulation Technique

The paravertebral space is located using an insulated 18-gauge Tuohy needle (continuous paravertebral technique) or a 22-gauge needle (single paravertebral block) connected to a nerve stimulator delivering a current of 2.5 to 5.0 mA with a pulse duration of 0.1 milliseconds and a frequency of 2 Hz.[43,67,68] When the insulated needle is at the proximity of the nerve bundle, a motor response is elicited (contraction of the intercostals or the abdominal muscle). This can result in an intercostal muscle contraction with

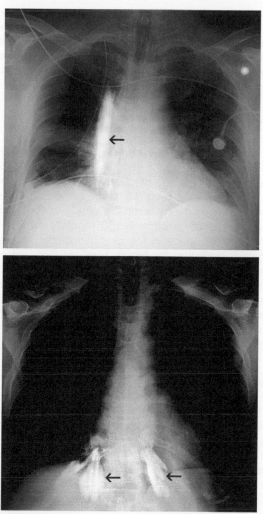

**Fig. 4.** Spread of the 10 mL of the contrast product demonstrating a paravertebral spread along the thoracic spine (as indicated by the *arrows*).

an intensity directly related to the distance between the needle and the intercostals nerve. The position of the needle is considered optimal when the muscle response is maintained with a current less than 0.5 mA.

## ULTRASOUND-GUIDED APPROACH

After determining the thoracic or lumbar level at which the block has to be performed, a parallel line 2.5 cm lateral to the spinous process, a low-frequency probe connected to an ultrasound machine, in our case an S-Nerve (Sonosite, Bothell, WA, USA), is applied parallel to the spinous process.[69–71] Scanning the area allows the identification of the transverse process, the costotransverse intercostalis ligament, the pleura, and the lung dynamically. This is facilitated by asking the patient to breathe deeply during the scanning. Using an in-plane approach, a needle is introduced between 2 corresponding transverse processes and positioned past the costotransverse inter-costals ligament and posterior to the parietal pleura. After negative aspiration for blood, 5 mL of local anesthetic is slowly injected. The injection of local anesthetic can be visualized, and the correct position of the needle is confirmed by seeing the local anesthetic volume pushing the pleura anteriorly. The anatomic landmarks are presented in **Figs. 1** and **2**.

## Lateral Approach to the Paravertebral Space

### Blind approach

The placement of a paravertebral catheter can be achieved using an intercostal approach (see **Fig. 3**). Depending on the segments to be blocked, the corresponding intercostal space is identified. The site of introduction of the needle is 8 cm from the corresponding spinous process. A 5-cm 18-gauge introducer Tuohy needle is intro-duced into the corresponding intercostal space initially to contact the rib. When the contact is established, the needle is reoriented 60° medially and at a 45° angle, pushed 1 cm within the intercostals space in the direction of the corresponding spinous process. After negative aspiration for blood, 5 mL of 0.5% ropivacaine is slowly injected to open the space. This is followed by the introduction of the catheter medially toward the corresponding paravertebral space. With such an approach it is expected that the catheter is positioned in the paravertebral space by traveling medially in the corresponding intercostal space. This approach offers the advantage of allowing access to the paravertebral space using a more superficial approach than the classic approach. This may be of some advantage to be safer, especially in patients with coagulopathy.

### Ultrasound-guided technique

The corresponding intercostal space is scanned by applying a 10- to 15-MHz probe 8 cm laterally from the spine to allow the identification of the ribs and pleura.[69,72] The identification of the pleura can be facilitated by asking the patient to breathe deeply and visualizing the movement of the lung. The probe is then rotated over the long axis of the rib and tilted to help identify the external intercostal muscle and internal intercostal membrane (**Figs. 5** and **6**). Lidocaine 1% is injected superficially at the site of introduction of the needle. The 18-gauge introducer Tuohy needle is introduced

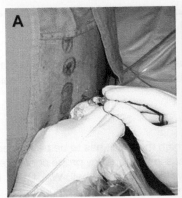 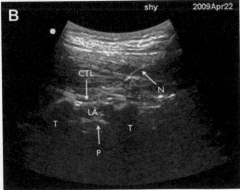

**Fig. 5.** Ultrasound approach to the paravertebral space. (*A*) Placement of the low-frequency probe and the needle. (*B*) Ultrasound image. CTL, costothoracic ligament; LA, local anes-thetics; N, needle; P, pleura; T, transverse process.

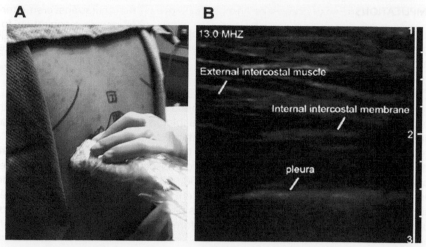

**Fig. 6.** Probe positioning (*A*) and ultrasound image (*B*) identifying the external intercostal muscle and internal intercostal membrane.

in plane and directed medially to position the tip of the needle between the internal intercostals membrane and the parietal pleura. After negative aspiration for blood, 5 mL of 5% ropivacaine is injected slowly. A 22-gauge catheter is introduced into the intercostal space and positioned 8 cm from the site of introduction of the needle. The introducer needle is removed and the catheter is secured in place using Steri-Strips. The catheter is protected by transparent dressing. After it is secured in place at the level of the corresponding surgery, an additional 10 mL of 0.5% ropivacaine is injected slowly after confirming negative aspiration for blood. This completes the block and also assures the patency of the paravertebral catheter.

## LOCAL ANESTHETIC MIXTURES AND MODE OF ADMINISTRATION

Bupivacaine, ropivacaine, and lidocaine have been the local anesthetics of choice to perform paravertebral blocks.[73] Although most practitioners do not recommend the use of additive, some recommend the addition of epinephrine, fentanyl, and clonidine to prolong the duration of the block. For single paravertebral blocks, the use of 0.50% (anesthesia) or 0.25% (analgesia) bupivacaine or 1.0% (anesthesia) or 0.5% (analgesia) ropivacaine has been advocated. In the case of continuous paravertebral blocks, 0.1 mL/kg of 0.5% bupivacaine and 1.0% lidocaine have been originally reported. At present, we favor the use of 0.2% ropivacaine, 0.06% bupivacaine, and 0.25% lidocaine starting at 7 mL/h per paravertebral catheter with a 3-mL bolus available per hour. This can be increased to 10 mL/h if necessary.

The effectiveness of this technique is significantly improved when the paravertebral block is part of a multimodal approach to pain management, including the use of ketamine 0.1 mg/kg intravenously followed by an infusion of 5 to 10 mg/h started in the recovery room. This can be combined with antiinflammatory drugs, such as ketorolac tromethamine (Toradol), 7.5 to 10 mg given intravenously every 6 hours for 48 hours, if there is no preexisting coagulopathy, allergy to nonsteroidal antiinflammatory drugs, or renal insufficiency. Such an approach can reduce the opioid requirements and opioid-related adverse events by 70% to 80%.

## COMPLICATIONS

It is established that the use of paravertebral blocks are safer than epidural and that complications with this technique are infrequent.[74,75] The most frequently reported complications are discussed.

### Pneumothorax and Pleural Puncture

Pleural puncture has been reported to occur around 1%, which may be reduced by the use of ultrasound guidance to perform these blocks. Pneumothorax is the most dreaded complication in the ambulatory setting and is estimated to occur at a frequency of around 0.5%. It is also reported that the performance of bilateral paravertebral blocks increases the potential for this complication by 8-fold. In the past few years that we have performed this block (over 30,000), we have had a total of 3 cases presenting with pneumothorax, with only 1 patient requiring the placement of a chest tube. The risk for pneumothorax exists in blocks performed between T1 and T8, and it is unlikely to occur in paravertebral blocks performed between T10 and L3.

### Bleeding

Hematoma following a paravertebral block has been reported to be around 2.4% and a risk of vascular puncture around 5%. Usually the hematoma is limited in magnitude. In performing continuous paravertebral blocks for thoracic surgery, we have observed bleeding of 50 mL or less in the chest in 1 patient. In this case, the aspiration of the blood revealed a vascular injury. When performing (**Fig. 7**) paravertebral blocks, it is possible to produce vascular injuries illustrated by the ability to aspirate blood via the needle during the procedure. Such an event is rare and certainly not associated with any major symptoms of development of significant hematoma.

### Epidural or Intrathecal Spread

This complication has been estimated to occur between 1% and 70%.[76,77] There are 3 factors that contribute to this. The first factor is the approach used with the needle. The investigators who reported up to 70% spread included those using an ultrasound-guided technique approach over the paravertebral space with a lateral to medial

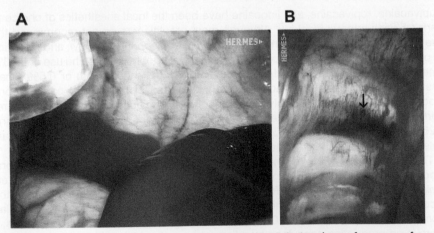

**Fig. 7.** Limited intrapleural bleed from a vascular puncture during the performance of a paravertebral block. (*A*) Blood in the chest cavity and (*B*) vascular puncture pointed out by the arrow.

needle direction, whereas those who reported infrequent epidural or intrathecal spread used a perpendicular approach parallel to the spinous process. Second, the volume of local anesthetics injected contributed to epidural spread. Most epidural spread occurred with volumes of 15 mL or higher. In the case of single paravertebral blocks, injecting 5 mL of the local anesthetic solution at multiple levels not only mini-mizes the risk for epidural spread but also provides a more extensive block. In the case of a continuous block, the initial injection of 5 mL of local anesthetic followed by injec-tion of 10 mL of local anesthetic through a multiorifice catheter also provided the optimum condition to avoid these side effects. In most cases, epidural spread is not associated with any significant clinical consequences except for transient hypoten-sion and bilateral lower limb weakness. The problem is more catastrophic when the needle is positioned intrathecally and is followed by an intrathecal injection of larger volume of the local anesthetic. When this occurs at a high thoracic level (T4 or higher), most of these patients required intubation and artificial ventilation until the effects of the injections dissipate. Third, practitioner inexperience and spinal deformity increase the risk of intrathecal administration of local anesthetics. This risk factor is greatly reduced when the block is performed using an ultrasound-guided technique. Irrespec-tive of the cause, injecting the local anesthetic slowly and fractionated represents an excellent technique to minimize the amount of local anesthetics injected intrathecally.

### Infection

Infection is a very rare complication. In our experience, we have not observed any abscess or systemic infection following the performance of a paravertebral block.[42] On rare occasions, we have observed a local infection/inflammation that did not require any treatment. The occurrence of this complication significantly correlates with the duration of the continuous block left in situ, similar to epidural analgesia.

### Nerve Injuries

As with any nerve block, performing paravertebral blocks can lead to occasional nerve injuries. Except for cervical and lumbar paravertebral blocks, injuries involved the sensory nerves and not motor nerves; therefore, the associated clinical symptoms included radiculopathy and pain similar to herpes zoster infection. The pain responds well to medications such as gabapentin (Neurontin) and pregabalin.

### Hypotension

Hypotension has been reported in 4% of cases. This is a much less frequent compli-cation than those reported when epidural is performed (30%). Hypotension could be attributed to the sympathetic blockade, epidural spread, or effect of local anesthetics on the vascular tone.

### Spinal Headache

Spinal headache occurs very infrequently.[78] Spinal headaches have been reported after the performance of paravertebral blocks. The most likely mechanism is trauma to the dural sleeve of the nerve in the paravertebral space during the performance of a paravertebral block that would lead to a leak of spinal fluid. In our experience, we recorded 2 cases of spinal headache.

## SUMMARY

Paravertebral block is one of the regional anesthesia techniques that has raised the most interest recently. The ongoing prospective studies on their role in delaying the recurrence of cancer and development of metastases will allow us to determine the role that this block can play in regional anesthesia.

## REFERENCES

1. Karmakar MK. Thoracic paravertebral block. Anesthesiology 2001;95(3):771–80.
2. Vila H Jr, Liu J, Kavasmaneck D. Paravertebral block: new benefits from an old procedure. Curr Opin Anaesthesiol 2007;20(4):316–8.
3. Exadaktylos AK, Buggy DJ, Moriarty DC, et al. Can anesthetic technique for primary breast cancer surgery affect recurrence or metastasis? Anesthesiology 2006;105(4):660–4.
4. Cheema SP, Ilsley D, Richardson J, et al. A thermographic study of paravertebral analgesia. Anaesthesia 1995;50(2):118–21.
5. Chelly JE, Uskova A, Merman R, et al. A multifactorial approach to the factors influencing determination of paravertebral depth. Can J Anaesth 2008;55(9): 587–94.
6. Choi S, Brull R. Neuraxial techniques in obstetric and non-obstetric patients with common bleeding diatheses. Anesth Analg 2009;109(2):648–60.
7. Klein SM, Nielsen KC, Ahmed N, et al. In situ images of the thoracic paravertebral space. Reg Anesth Pain Med 2004;29(6):596–9.
8. Naja MZ, Gustafsson AC, Ziade MF, et al. Distance between the skin and the thoracic paravertebral space. Anaesthesia 2005;60(7):680–4.
9. Thavaneswaran P, Rudkin GE, Cooter RD, et al. Brief reports: paravertebral block for anesthesia: a systematic review. Anesth Analg 2010;110(6):1740–4.
10. Buckenmaier CC 3rd, Steele SM, Nielsen KC, et al. Bilateral continuous paravertebral catheters for reduction mammoplasty. Acta Anaesthesiol Scand 2002; 46(8):1042–5.
11. Buggy DJ, Kerin MJ. Paravertebral analgesia with levobupivacaine increases postoperative flap tissue oxygen tension after immediate latissimus dorsi breast reconstruction compared with intravenous opioid analgesia. Anesthesiology 2004;100(2):375–80.
12. Cooter RD, Rudkin GE, Gardiner SE. Day case breast augmentation under paravertebral blockade: a prospective study of 100 consecutive patients. Aesthetic Plast Surg 2007;31(6):666–73.
13. Greengrass R, O'Brien F, Lyerly K, et al. Paravertebral block for breast cancer surgery. Can J Anaesth 1996;43(8):858–61.
14. Pusch F, Freitag H, Weinstabl C, et al. Single-injection paravertebral block compared to general anaesthesia in breast surgery. Acta Anaesthesiol Scand 1999;43(7):770–4.
15. Sopena-Zubiria LA, Fernández-Meré LA, Muñoz González F, et al. [Multiple-injection thoracic paravertebral block for reconstructive breast surgery]. Rev Esp Anestesiol Reanim 2010;57(6):357–63 [in Spanish].
16. Greengrass R, Buckenmaier CC 3rd. Paravertebral anaesthesia/analgesia for ambulatory surgery. Best Pract Res Clin Anaesthesiol 2002;16(2):271–83.
17. Hadzic A, Kerimoglu B, Loreio D, et al. Paravertebral blocks provide superior same-day recovery over general anesthesia for patients undergoing inguinal hernia repair. Anesth Analg 2006;102(4):1076–81.
18. Klein SM, Greengrass RA, Weltz C, et al. Paravertebral somatic nerve block for outpatient inguinal herniorrhaphy: an expanded case report of 22 patients. Reg Anesth Pain Med 1998;23(3):306–10.
19. Jamieson BD, Mariano ER. Thoracic and lumbar paravertebral blocks for outpatient lithotripsy. J Clin Anesth 2007;19(2):149–51.

20. Johansson A, Renck H, Aspelin P, et al. Multiple intercostal blocks by a single injection? A clinical and radiological investigation. Acta Anaesthesiol Scand 1985;29(5):524–8.

21. Chaudakshetrin P, Ketuman P. Anesthetic pain management in Siriraj Hospital: a retrospective review. J Med Assoc Thai 2002;85(Suppl 3):S858–65.

22. Gerner P. Post-thoracotomy pain management problems. Anesthesiol Clin 2008; 26(2):355–67.

23. Gilbert J, Hultman J. Thoracic paravertebral block: a method of pain control. Acta Anaesthesiol Scand 1989;33:142–5.

24. Gottschalk A, Cohen SP, Yang S, et al. Preventing and treating pain after thoracic surgery. Anesthesiology 2006;104(3):594–600.

25. Lee EM, Murphy KP, Ben-David B. Postoperative analgesia for hip arthroscopy: combined L1 and L2 paravertebral blocks. J Clin Anesth 2008;20(6):462–5.

26. Basagan-Mogol E, Turker G, Yilmaz M, et al. Combination of a psoas compartment, sciatic nerve, and T12-L1 paravertebral blocks for femoropopliteal bypass surgery in a high-risk patient. J Cardiothorac Vasc Anesth 2008; 22(2):337–9.

27. Ganapathy S, Nielsen KC, Steele SM. Outcomes after paravertebral blocks. Int Anesthesiol Clin 2005;43(3):185–93.

28. Olivier JF, Bracco D, Nguyen P, et al. Perioperative Cardiac Surgery Research Group (PeriCARG). A novel approach for pain management in cardiac surgery via median sternotomy: bilateral single-shot paravertebral blocks. Heart Surg Forum 2007;10(5):E357–62.

29. Tsai T, Rodriguez-Diaz C, Deschner B, et al. Thoracic paravertebral block for implantable cardioverter-defibrillator and laser lead extraction. J Clin Anesth 2008;20(5):379–82.

30. Ben-David B, Swanson J, Nelson JB, et al. Multimodal analgesia for radical prostatectomy provides better analgesia and shortens hospital stay. J Clin Anesth 2007;19(4):264–8.

31. Perttunen K, Nilsson E, Heinonen J, et al. Extradural, paravertebral and intercostal nerve blocks for post-thoracotomy pain. Br J Anaesth 1995;75(5):541–7.

32. Purcell-Jones G, Justins DM. Postoperative paravertebral blocks for thoracic surgery. Br J Anaesth 1988;61(3):369–70.

33. Richardson J, Sabanathan S, Mearns AJ, et al. A prospective, randomized comparison of interpleural and paravertebral analgesia in thoracic surgery. Br J Anaesth 1995;75:405–8.

34. Burns DA, Ben-David B, Chelly JE, et al. Blockade. Anesth Analg 2008;107(1): 339–41.

35. Culp WC Jr, Culp WC. Thoracic paravertebral block for percutaneous transhepatic biliary drainage. J Vasc Interv Radiol 2005;16(10):1397–400.

36. Culp WC, McCowan TC, DeValdenebro M, et al. Paravertebral block: an improved method of pain control in percutaneous transhepatic biliary drainage. Cardiovasc Intervent Radiol 2006;29(6):1015–21.

37. Finnerty O, Carney J, McDonnell JG. Trunk blocks for abdominal surgery. Anaesthesia 2010;65(Suppl 1):76–83.

38. Hill SE, Keller RA, Stafford-Smith M, et al. Efficacy of single-dose, multilevel paravertebral nerve blockade for analgesia after thoracoscopic procedures. Anesthesiology 2006;104(5):1047–53.

39. Joshi GP, Bonnet F, Shah R, et al. A systematic review of randomized trials evaluating regional techniques for post-thoracotomy analgesia. Anesth Analg 2008; 107:1026–40.

40. Kaya FN, Turker G, Basagan-Mogol E, et al. Preoperative multiple-injection thoracic paravertebral blocks reduce postoperative pain and analgesic requirements after video-assisted thoracic surgery. J Cardiothorac Vasc Anesth 2006; 20(5):639–43.

41. Tacconi F, Pompeo E, Fabbi E, et al. Awake video-assisted pleural decortication for empyema thoracis. Eur J Cardiothorac Surg 2010;37(3):594–601.

42. Adelman H, Milton M, Irwin I, et al. Acute aseptic meningitis following paravertebral lumbar sympathetic blocks. Anesthesiology 1946;7(4):422–5.

43. Boezaart AP, Lucas SD, Elliott CE. Paravertebral block: cervical, thoracic, lumbar, and sacral. Curr Opin Anaesthesiol 2009;22(5):637–43.

44. Buckenmaier CC 3rd, Steele SM, Nielsen KC, et al. Paravertebral somatic nerve blocks for breast surgery in a patient with hypertrophic obstructive cardiomyopathy. Can J Anaesth 2002;49(6):571–4.

45. Català E, Casas JI, Unzueta MC, et al. Continuous infusion is superior to bolus doses with thoracic paravertebral blocks after thoracotomies. J Cardiothorac Vasc Anesth 1996;10(5):586–8.

46. Daly DJ, Myles PS. Update on the role of paravertebral blocks for thoracic surgery: are they worth it? Curr Opin Anaesthesiol 2009;22(1):38–43.

47. De Cosmo G, Aceto P, Gualtieri E, et al. Analgesia in thoracic surgery: review. Minerva Anestesiol 2009;75(6):393–400.

48. Richardson J, Sabanathan S, Shah R. Post-thoracotomy spirometric lung function: the effect of analgesia. A review. J Cardiovasc Surg (Torino) 1999;40(3): 445–56.

49. Tenicela R, Pollan SB. Paravertebral-peridural block technique: a unilateral thoracic block [review]. Clin J Pain 1990;6(3):227–34.

50. Burton AW, Eappen S. Regional anesthesia techniques for pain control in the intensive care unit. Crit Care Clin 1999;15(1):77–88.

51. Karmakar MK, Chui PT, Joynt GM, et al. Thoracic paravertebral block for management of pain associated with multiple fractured ribs in patients with concomitant lumbar spinal trauma. Reg Anesth Pain Med 2001;26:169–73.

52. Karmakar MK, Ho AM. Acute pain management of patients with multiple fractured ribs. J Trauma 2003;54:615–25.

53. Antila H, Kirvelä O. Neurolytic thoracic paravertebral block in cancer pain. A clinical report. Acta Anaesthesiol Scand 1998;42(5):581–5.

54. Chaturvedi A, Dash HH. Sympathetic blockade for the relief of chronic pain. J Indian Med Assoc 2001;99(12):698–703.

55. Clark JM. Paravertebral C2 nerve blocks. Headache 1995;35(7):437.

56. Conacher ID, Kokri M. Postoperative paravertebral blocks for thoracic surgery. A radiological appraisal. Br J Anaesth 1987;59(2):155–61.

57. Esch AT, Esch A, Knorr JL, et al. Long-term ambulatory continuous nerve blocks for terminally ill patients: a case series. Pain Med 2010;11(8):1299–302.

58. Kirvelä O, Antila H. Thoracic paravertebral block in chronic postoperative pain. Reg Anesth 1992;17(6):348–50.

59. Nikiforov S, Cronin AJ, Murray WB, et al. Subcutaneous paravertebral block for renal colic. Anesthesiology 2001;94(3):531.

60. Ohtori S, Yamashita M, Inoue G, et al. L2 spinal nerve-block effects on acute low back pain from osteoporotic vertebral fracture. J Pain 2009;10(8):870–5.

61. Paniagua P, Català E, Villar Landeira JM. Successful management of pleuritic pain with thoracic paravertebral block. Reg Anesth Pain Med 2000;25(6):651–3.

62. Pedersen JL, Rung GW, Kehlet H. Effect of sympathetic nerve block on acute inflammatory pain and hyperalgesia. Anesthesiology 1997;86(2):293–301.

63. Nair V, Henry R. Bilateral paravertebral block: a satisfactory alternative for labour analgesia. Can J Anaesth 2001;48(2):179–84.
64. Naja Z, Lönnqvist PA. Somatic paravertebral nerve blockade. Incidence of failed block and complications. Anaesthesia 2001;56(12):1184–8.
65. Suelto MD. Paravertebral lumbar sympathetic block for labor analgesia. Anesthesiology 2000;93(2):580.
66. Richardson J, Cheema SP, Hawkins J, et al. Thoracic paravertebral space location. A new method using pressure measurement. Anaesthesia 1996;51(2):137–9.
67. Boezaart AP, De Beer JF, Nell ML. Early experience with continuous cervical paravertebral block using a stimulating catheter. Reg Anesth Pain Med 2003;28(5):406–13.
68. Lang SA. The use of a nerve stimulator or thoracic paravertebral block. Anesthesiology 2002;97(2):521.
69. Abrahams MS, Horn JL, Noles LM, et al. Evidence-based medicine: ultrasound guidance for truncal blocks. Reg Anesth Pain Med 2010;35(Suppl 2):S36–42.
70. Tsui B, Suresh S. Ultrasound imaging for regional anesthesia in infants, children, and adolescents: a review of current literature and its application in the practice of extremity and trunk blocks. Anesthesiology 2010;112(2):473–92.
71. Tsui BC, Suresh S. Ultrasound imaging for regional anesthesia in infants, children, and adolescents: a review of current literature and its application in the practice of neuraxial blocks. Anesthesiology 2010;112(3):719–28.
72. Pusch F, Wildling E, Klimscha W, et al. Sonographic measurement of needle insertion depth in paravertebral blocks in women. Br J Anaesth 2000;85(6):841–3.
73. Karmakar MK, Ho AM, Law BK, et al. Arterial and venous pharmacokinetics of ropivacaine with and without epinephrine after thoracic paravertebral block. Anesthesiology 2005;103(4):704–11.
74. Lönnqvist PA, MacKenzie J, Soni AK, et al. Paravertebral blockade. Failure rate and complications. Anaesthesia 1995;50(9):813–5.
75. Ohseto K. Efficacy of thoracic sympathetic ganglion block and prediction of complications: clinical evaluation of the anterior paratracheal and posterior paravertebral approaches in 234 patients. J Anesth 1992;6(3):316–31.
76. Frohm RM, Raw RM, Haider N, et al. Epidural spread after continuous cervical paravertebral block: a case report. Reg Anesth Pain Med 2006;31(3):279–81.
77. Garutti I, Hervias M, Barrio JM, et al. Subdural spread of local anesthetic agent following thoracic paravertebral block and cannulation. Anesthesiology 2003;98(4):1005–7.
78. Lin HM, Chelly JE. Post-dural headache associated with thoracic paravertebral blocks. J Clin Anesth 2006;18(5):376–8.
79. Casati A, Alessandrini P, Nuzzi M, et al. Prospective, randomized, blinded comparison between continuous thoracic paravertebral and epidural infusion of 0.2% ropivacaine after lung resection surgery. Eur J Anaesthesiol 2006;23:999–1004.
80. Davies RG, Myles PS, Graham JM. A comparison of the analgesic efficacy and side-effects of paravertebral vs. epidural blockade for thoracotomy—a systematic review and meta-analysis of randomized trials. Br J Anaesth 2006;96:418–26.
81. Dhole S, Mehta Y, Saxena H, et al. Comparison of continuous thoracic epidural and paravertebral blocks for postoperative analgesia after minimally invasive direct coronary artery bypass surgery. J Cardiothorac Vasc Anesth 2001;15(3):288–92.

82. Frank SM, El-Rahmany HK, Tran KM, et al. Comparison of lower extremity cutaneous temperature changes in patients receiving lumbar sympathetic ganglion blocks versus epidural anesthesia. J Clin Anesth 2000;12(7):525–30.
83. Richardson J, Sabanathan S, Jones J, et al. A prospective, randomized comparison of preoperative and continuous balanced epidural or paravertebral bupivacaine on post-thoracotomy pain, pulmonary function and stress responses. Br J Anaesth 1999;83(3):387–92.
84. Scarci M, Joshi A, Attia R. In patients undergoing thoracic surgery is paravertebral block as effective as epidural analgesia for pain management? Interact Cardiovasc Thorac Surg 2010;10:92–6.

# Recent Advances in Multimodal Analgesia

Adam Young, MD, Asokumar Buvanendran, MD*

KEYWORDS

- Injectable acetaminophen and ibuprofen
- Topical NSAIDs for multimodal analgesia • Capsaicin
- Tapentadol • Depot formulation of local anesthetic

Multimodal analgesia captures the effectiveness of individual agents in optimal dosages that maximize efficacy and attempts to minimize side effects from one analgesic. This important concept uses the theory that agents with different mechanisms of analgesia that may have synergistic effects in preventing or treating acute pain when used in combination. These regimens must be tailored to individual patients, keeping in mind the procedure being performed, side effects of individual medications, and patients' preexisting medical conditions.[1] The concept and theory of multimodal analgesia is not new; however, several novel pharmacologic agents have emerged and can be added to the drugs that can be used in this manner. It is vital to realize that blocking the neuronal pathway during surgery with local anesthetics does not decrease the humeral biochemical responses that occur during surgery, which have to be inhibited by administering systemic pharmacologic therapy.[2] This review focuses on the recent advances in pharmacologic agents for multimodal therapy.

## ACETAMINOPHEN

Oral acetaminophen has been used for several decades and believed to have a central role of action in analgesia because of its antipyretic properties and confers several mild analgesia antiinflammatory properties.[3] Paracetamol, an intravenous (IV) formulation of acetaminophen, became available in 2002 and has been studied in Europe. Göröcs and colleagues[4] administered a single dose of 1 g of IV paracetamol (Perfalgan) before the termination of surgery and observed high patient satisfaction and good tolerance of the drug in 601 patients undergoing minor outpatient surgical procedures. Nearly half of these patients (42.7%) received the lone dose of

No funding was obtained to write this article.

Department of Anesthesiology, Rush University Medical Center, 1653 West Congress Parkway, 763 Jelke, Chicago, IL 60612, USA

* Corresponding author.

E-mail address: Asokumar@aol.com

paracetamol as monotherapy for postoperative pain. Salihoglu and colleagues[5] randomized 40 patients undergoing laparoscopic cholecystectomy to 1 g paracetamol (after intubation and before incision) or saline infusion. Significant improvements in outcomes in the paracetamol group included lower visual analog score (VAS), lower morphine consumption, and shorter stay in the recovery room (32 ± 11 vs 48 ± 14 minutes). Approved by the US Food and Drug Administration (FDA) in November 2010, IV acetaminophen (Ofirmev) has been studied and shown to be safe. IV acetaminophen endorses a quick onset with meaningful pain relief achieved 25 minutes after administration in patients undergoing laparoscopic surgery,[6] 25 to 27 minutes after total hip arthroplasty.[7] Ender and colleagues[8] retrospectively evaluated the use of a fast-track protocol (which included IV acetaminophen) for cardiac surgery in 421 patients compared with matched controls who were not fast-tracked and did not receive IV acetaminophen. Acetaminophen was administered, 1 g every 6 hours, postoperatively. Significant results included shorter times to extubation (75 vs 90 minutes), shorter intensive care units stays (4 vs 20 hours), shorter intermediate stays (21 vs 26 hours), and shorter hospital stay (10 vs 11 days). The ability of these compounds to shorten hospital stays, while providing safe and effective analgesia, should garner the attention of not only anesthesiologists but also hospital administrators keen on cost-effective care. The oral administration of acetaminophen can probably achieve the same results as IV acetaminophen in patients who have a functioning gastrointestinal system. However, it is also to be noted that the analgesic effect is much more rapid than oral because of the pharmacokinetics.

As based on current research, combinations of acetaminophen and nonsteroidal antiinflammatory drugs (NSAIDs) have been investigated and may offer enhanced effects. In 55 children undergoing hernia repair, 30-mg ketorolac and 20-mg/kg acetaminophen resulted in significantly lower postoperative fentanyl consumption and less sedation and vomiting.[9] A systematic review of this subject determined that when used as a combination, NSAIDs and paracetamol "offer superior analgesia compared with either drug alone,"[10] and 18 of 21 studies included had positive results with regard to lowering VAS and/or use of rescue analgesics. The combination was more effective than paracetamol (85% of studies) or NSAIDs (64% of studies) alone.

## NSAIDs

The use of NSAID in the perioperative period has been well established taking into consideration the adverse effects of bleeding. The utility of cyclooxygenase 2 inhibitors in this scenario has been demonstrated to be a benefit.[1,2] A randomized, double-blind, placebo-controlled study comparing celecoxib, 200 mg, with placebo in 37 patients undergoing major plastic surgery demonstrated the ability of celecoxib to reduce VAS and postoperative morphine consumption. More importantly, the treatment groups had earlier return of bowel function (2 vs 3 days), resumed normal physical activities earlier (4 vs 6 days), and had higher patient satisfaction scores.[11]

More recent formulations of NSAIDs include intranasal (IN) ketorolac spray, IV ibuprofen, and topical diclofenac. Southworth and colleagues[12] conducted a randomized double-blind trial of varying dosages of IV ibuprofen (Caldolor) versus placebo in 406 patients who underwent an elective abdominal or orthopedic surgery. Those receiving ibuprofen, 800 mg every 6 hours, consumed 22% less morphine postoperatively. IV ibuprofen, 400 mg every 6 hours, seemed to attenuate postoperative pain for up to 24 hours but had no benefit thereafter when compared with placebo. Aside from dizziness, IV ibuprofen was generally well tolerated.

In a randomized, double-blind, placebo-controlled study comparing IN ketorolac with placebo in 40 patients undergoing third molar extraction, Grant and Mehlisch[13] demonstrated that 31.5-mg IN ketorolac resulted in higher pain relief scores and greater patient satisfaction. Sixty percent of participants in the study group reported good to excellent pain control compared with 13% in the placebo group. IN ketorolac, 31.5 mg every 6 hours for 48 hours and then up to 4 times daily (up to 5 days), in patients undergoing abdominal surgery decreased morphine use over 48 hours and resulted in a higher quality of analgesia scores.[14] The investigators of this study indicated that pain relief occurred within 20 minutes of administration, which may be because of higher blood-brain penetration of ketorolac via the nasal route (cribriform plate). The availability of IN ketorolac can now be used in the ambulatory setting after discharge from hospital, taking the same general precautions as IV formulation.

Topical diclofenac exists in several forms, including diclofenac epolamine 1% topical patch (FLECTOR Patch), diclofenac sodium 1% topical gel (VOLTAREN Gel), and diclofenac sodium 1.5% w/w liquid (PENNSAID). A thorough review by Massey and colleagues[15] showed that topical NSAIDs are not only safe but also efficacious in the treatment of acute soft tissue injuries and localized regions of pain, acute or chronic. The investigators did find a difference between placebo and topical NSAIDs with regard to local skin irritation, but the systemic side effects were less with topical NSAIDs. In fact, most current research point to the fact that topical application of diclofenac could lead to decreased systemic absorption and therefore less gastrointestinal and renal adverse events associated with this class of drug. This research has even led to the National Institute for Health and Clinical Excellence (UK) to recommend topical NSAIDs, along with acetaminophen, as first-line treatment of osteoarthritis pain.[16]

A review of diclofenac epolamine topical patch by McCarberg and Argoff[17] discussed the benefits of a patch, as opposed to NSAID gels or creams. These benefits included application of a defined dose of diclofenac, drug delivery over an extended period of time (typically 12 hours), and ease of application. Barthel and colleagues[18] investigated the application of diclofenac sodium 1% gel versus placebo vehicle (identical composition to the gel component of the study drug) applied 4 times daily for 3 months for the treatment of osteoarthritis pain. Results of their study indicated superior analgesia from 1 to 12 weeks and improved function for the same duration. Diclofenac gel was tolerated as well as placebo. With regard to diclofenac 1.5% w/w liquid, the gel has been shown to be as efficacious as oral diclofenac in treating arthritis pain.[19] Gastrointestinal side effects were significantly less common, with local skin reactions being more common. A prospective study by Shainhouse and colleagues[20] established the safety of topical diclofenac 1.5% w/w in a study in which 793 subjects were followed up for an average of 204 days; 144 subjects were followed up for 1 year. Application of the study drug, 40 drops 4 times daily, resulted in local skin reactions (dry skin, contact dermatitis, or dermatitis with vesicles) in 45.1% of study participants. Twenty-four volunteers indicated a similar overall experience when using diclofenac gel and diclofenac liquid. However, the investigators found the gel to have a less desirable scent and found the consistency to be more greasy and sticky than the diclofenac liquid.[21] When side effects have limited oral NSAID use in a multimodal analgesia, it may be that IN, IV, and topical formulations of NSAIDs could prove to be of benefit in the perioperative period and should be considered as tools that are emerging for multimodal analgesia.

## ANTICONVULSANTS

The use of adjunct agents to treat pain includes the use of anticonvulsants such as gabapentin and pregabalin. Clarke and colleagues[22] studied the effects of varying doses of gabapentin given preoperatively and postoperatively in addition to femoral/sciatic nerve blocks and celecoxib in 36 patients undergoing total knee arthroplasty. When administered preoperatively and postoperatively, gabapentin decreased morphine consumption on postoperative days (PODs) 2 to 4 and increased the amount of active knee flexion on PODs 2 to 3. This occurred without an increase in side effects. A randomized, double-blind, controlled trial of gabapentin in children undergoing spinal fusion determined that preoperative and postoperative gabapentin resulted in decreased morphine consumption and improved pain scores through the early stages of recovery up to POD 2.[23] However, this attenuation of opioid use and decreased verbal pain scores were temporary. An evaluation of gabapentin's ability to prevent not only acute but also chronic pain by Sen and colleagues[24] revealed that gabapentin, 1200 mg, administered preoperatively decreased morphine consumption; reduced incisional pain at 1, 3, and 6 months; and improved patient satisfaction when compared with placebo. Comparing varying dosages of gabapentin in lumbar laminectomy, Khan and colleagues[25] concluded that the timing of dosing (preoperative vs postoperative) did not affect analgesic efficacy. Gabapentin administered, 900 mg or 1200 mg preoperatively or postoperatively, reduced morphine consumption in the first 24 hours after operation and VAS scores without increase in side effects.

The use of a similar anticonvulsant, pregabalin, has gained attention because of more favorable pharmacokinetics, which includes improved bioavailability and faster achievement of therapeutic levels. Thirty patients undergoing laparoscopic cholecystectomy were randomized to receive pregabalin, 150 mg 1 hour preoperatively, or placebo by Agarwal and colleagues.[26] Fentanyl use and VAS scores were measured up to 24 hours postoperatively. Both VAS scores and narcotic use were significantly lower in patients who had received pregabalin. No significant difference in side effects was noted. Mathiesen and colleagues[27] studied a single preoperative dose of pregabalin, 300 mg, versus pregabalin, 300 mg, plus dexamethasone, 8 mg, in 120 patients undergoing total hip arthroplasty. Although pain scores were unaffected, the 2 groups receiving pregabalin preoperatively had significantly less morphine consumption at 24 hours postoperation. The investigators did notice that those receiving pregabalin had more sedation. A randomized, placebo-controlled, double-blind trial comparing pregabalin (300 mg preoperatively with a tapering dose postoperatively for 14 days) with placebo in 240 patients undergoing total knee arthroplasty has recently been published.[28] Immediate effects observed were decreased epidural drug consumption and increased sedation and confusion on PODs 0 and 1. Long-term outcomes included reduced neuropathic pain at 3 and 6 months. A meta-analysis by Zhang and colleagues[29] demonstrated that pregabalin administered preoperatively and/or postoperatively decreases 24-hour morphine consumption while having no effect on postoperative pain scales. Analysis also revealed that pregabalin administration led to lower rates of postoperative nausea and vomiting. The only significant side effect observed was visual disturbances with trends toward more sedation and dizziness/headache in pregabalin-treated groups. This meta-analysis did not include any studies of prolonged (more than 2) doses of pregabalin.

### TRPV1 AGONIST: CAPSAICIN

Capsaicin, the active component of chili peppers, selectively stimulates unmyelinated C fiber afferent neurons and causes the release of substance P. After initial depolarization, continued release of substance P in the presence of capsaicin leads to the depletion of substance P and subsequent decrease in C fiber activation. Capsaicin is a nonnarcotic that acts at TRPV1 receptor as an agonist peripherally. It does not affect the A delta and A alpha fibers. Capsaicin causes calcium-dependent desensitization.

An ultrapurified capsaicin (ALGRX 4975, 98% pure) has been investigated in a randomized, double-blind, placebo-controlled study on the analgesic efficacy of a single intraoperative wound instillation of 1000 µg of capsaicin after open mesh groin hernia repair.[30] The VAS pain scores assessed as area under the curve was significantly lower during the first 3 days postoperatively, but this effect was not observed after 72 hours. The local application of capsaicin during hernia repair does not lead to loss of sensory function in patients[31] and has been demonstrated in animal studies not to cause neurotoxicity.[32] Further clinical trials have been performed in patients undergoing total knee and hip arthroplasty, but the entire data have not been published to date. When capsaicin is used in the perioperative setting, the clinician must administer capsaicin well before the end of anesthesia to allow for resolution of the acute burning sensation that occurs immediately after its application. The prolonged duration of analgesia obtained by capsaicin could be extremely valuable in facilitating earlier rehabilitation after painful orthopedic surgery procedures. In contrast to local anesthetics, capsaicin does not affect the motor or autonomic functions and therefore does not interfere with postoperative rehabilitation. The capsaicin patch (NGX-4010), although used for various neuropathic chronic pain conditions, may be useful in acute pain in a multimodal manner. This needs further large-scale randomized controlled trials.

## N-METHYL-D-ASPARTATE RECEPTOR ANTAGONISTS

N-methyl-D-aspartate (NMDA) receptor antagonists, including ketamine and memantine, have been studied as adjuncts for acute and chronic pain management. Ketamine has options for routes of administration, including IV or IN. Remérand and colleagues[33] demonstrated that an IV bolus at the beginning of surgery followed by a 24-hour infusion decreased morphine consumption in patients undergoing total hip arthroplasty. Also, in patients receiving ketamine, the incidence of chronic pain was decreased. At 6 months, 21% of placebo and 8% of ketamine-receiving patients had persistent pain. Loftus and colleagues[34] found similar results, albeit in opiate-dependent patients undergoing lumbar spine surgery. A ketamine infusion of 10 µg/kg/min was started at the beginning of surgery after a bolus of 0.5 mg/kg was administered and terminated at skin closure. Significant results included decreased postoperative morphine requirements and lower pain scores at 6 weeks after operation.

Memantine was first synthesized in the 1960s and found to antagonize the NMDA receptor in the 1980s. The major site of action is the blockade of current flow through the NMDA receptor channel. Memantine is completely absorbed from the gastrointestinal tract, with maximal plasma concentration occurring between 3 and 8 hours after oral administration. Food does not influence the bioavailability of memantine. Approximately 80% of the administered dose remains as the parent drug. The mean terminal elimination half-life is 60 to 100 hours. The recommended initial dose of memantine hydrochloride for the treatment of moderate to severe dementia of Alzheimer disease type is 5 mg orally once daily. The dose should be increased in 5-mg increments to 10 mg/d. The minimum recommended interval between dose increases is 1 week. The recommended maintenance dose is 10 mg twice daily (20 mg/d). There is not an established dose for the treatment of chronic pain states, but case reports and medication trials that have started at 5 to 10 mg twice a day with increases at 1-week intervals to 30 mg/d have been examined. Ketamine causes memory deficits, reproduces with impressive accuracy the symptoms of schizophrenia, is widely abused, and induces vacuoles in neurons at moderate concentrations and cell death at higher concentrations. Memantine, on the other hand, is well tolerated; although instances of psychotic side effects have been reported, in placebo-controlled clinical studies the incidence of side effects is remarkably low.

Memantine, an orally administered noncompetitive NMDA receptor antagonist, may prove to be more useful than ketamine as an analgesia adjunct. In one study, daily doses of memantine, 30 mg, decreased phantom pain by up to 80% at 1 month after upper extremity amputations (in combination with brachial plexus block.)[35] However, in patients who have developed phantom pain, the pain relief obtained is temporary. Once chronic pain from surgery is established, such as phantom limb pain, memantine has not been shown to provide analgesia for these patients.

Magnesium seems to exert its analgesic mechanism via inhibition of calcium influx, antagonism of NMDA receptors, and prevention of enhanced ligand-induced NMDA signaling in a state of hypomagnesemia. In addition, magnesium may attenuate central sensitization after peripheral tissue injury or inflammation because of dorsal horn NMDA receptors. Magnesium sulfate is available as a 500-mg/mL preservative-free solution for injection. Magnesium administered intravenously lacks efficacy at 4 g; however, 50 mg administered intrathecally has been demonstrated to be effective.[36] Perioperative IV magnesium sulfate at very high doses has been reported to reduce postoperative morphine consumption but not postoperative pain scores. A dose-finding study for IV magnesium determined that administration of magnesium at 40 mg/kg before induction, followed by a 10-mg/kg/h infusion, resulted in a reduction in perioperative analgesic requirements without any major hemodynamic consequences.[37] Higher infusion doses did not offer any advantage. However, because the magnesium ion poorly crosses the blood-brain barrier in humans, it is not clear whether the therapeutic effect is related to NMDA antagonism in the central or peripheral nervous system. This needs to be investigated further.

## $\alpha_2$ AGONISTS

Use of $\alpha_2$ agonists as an analgesia adjunct has gained interest with clonidine and dexmedetomidine. Central and peripheral stimulation of the $\alpha_2$ receptors is believed to be the basic mechanism behind analgesia. The role of clonidine in neuraxial blockade has been described by several studies. Recently, Lena and colleagues[38] compared a clonidine/morphine spinal plus remifentanil infusion with a sufentanil infusion for analgesia in 83 patients undergoing open heart surgery. The clonidine/morphine spinal group had faster times to extubation and lower pain scores postoperatively, used less patient-controlled analgesia (PCA) morphine, and had improved patient satisfaction.

An infusion of dexmedetomidine, administered before induction through wound closure, decreased postanesthesia care unit (PACU) opioid use in 80 patients undergoing laparoscopic bariatric surgery.[39] In addition to this, nausea and vomiting was decreased and PACU stay shortened. As presumed, higher doses of dexmedetomidine required significantly more rescue doses of phenylephrine intraoperatively, otherwise there were no differences in side effects compared with placebo. Ramadhyani and colleagues[40] reviewed the use of dexmedetomidine in IV regional anesthesia. The investigators concluded that when added to IV regional solutions, dexmedetomidine had the ability to prolong analgesia and extend the duration of motor and sensory blockade.

## DUAL-ACTING AGENT: TAPENTADOL

Tapentadol is a novel central-acting analgesic with duel mode of action.[41] It has analgesic action via the μ opioid receptor and norepinephrine reuptake inhibition. Combining both effects in a single molecule eliminates the potential for drug-drug interactions inherent in multiple drug therapy. The analgesic effects of tapentadol are independent of metabolic activation with minimal metabolites. Having limited protein binding, no active metabolites, and no significant microsomal enzyme induction or inhibition, tapentadol has a limited potential for drug-drug interactions. The duel mode of analgesia is synergistic as demonstrated by preclinical work. The immediate release formulation of tapentadol is FDA approved and has been used in the United States since 2008 with 50, 75, and 100 mg. The drug is a Schedule II drug, and, as such, all precautions that need to be followed for other drugs in this category needs to be followed. The equipotent analgesic dose of 100 mg of tapentadol to oxycodone is 15 mg and needs to be administered 4 to 6 hours.

Although this compound has opioid activity, it also has activity at the descending pathway and therefore may prove to be a very useful analgesic as more clinical experience is obtained in the postoperative setting. For equipotent doses of narcotics, tapentadol has decreased incidence of nausea and vomiting compared with oxycodone.[42] The concept of obtaining equipotent analgesia with decreased postoperative nausea and vomiting can be of great benefit in treating postoperative pain and earlier discharge with significant cost savings.[43] However, further clinical trials need to be performed to demonstrate this phenomenon.

## EMERGING TECHNOLOGIES IN PAIN MANAGEMENT
### Transdermal Fentanyl

The use of patient-controlled delivery has led to the development of other modalities that allow patient control in the delivery of opioid medications. Transdermal delivery systems, such as IONSYS, allow demand dosing of fentanyl at a predetermined interval. The fentanyl hydrochloride iontophoretic transdermal system (ITS) is a patient-controlled approach to analgesic delivery that may avoid some of the problems associated with IV PCA. Fentanyl ITS is a compact, needleless, self-contained system that is preprogrammed to deliver fentanyl, 40 μg, across the skin by means of an imperceptible low-intensity electrical current, a method known as iontophoresis. This needleless system is under further research before being released for human use. Inhaled fentanyl has been trialed in pediatric and adult patients. There are investigations into the encapsulated liposomal inhaled fentanyl for acute pain, the advantage of this being that it can provide rapid onset and sustained release.

### Long-Acting Local Anesthetics

A newly developed liposomal long-acting bupivacaine is considered for approval by the FDA. A single injection of the liposomal bupivacaine should last 72 hours and is currently considered for infiltration of the local surgical site. Regional analgesia with this product has yet to be established.

### Cannabinoids

These compounds have been shown to be potent analgesics in animal models. There have been several clinical trials, most of them demonstrating no significant analgesic effect superior to placebo.[44] In fact, some of the trials demonstrated increase in VAS with nabilone (oral synthetic cannabinoid) when used in acute postoperative setting. However, these classes of drugs seem to be promising in patients with chronic pain.

## SUMMARY

Acute postoperative pain is a predictable response. Recent research has demonstrated that untreated acute postoperative pain can lead to chronic persistent pain. It is imperative that the health care provider managing acute postoperative pain understand the various options such as multimodal analgesia so that acute pain can be treated and development of chronic pain from surgery prevented.

## REFERENCES

1. Buvanendran A, Kroin JS. Multimodal analgesia for controlling acute postoperative pain. Curr Opin Anaesthesiol 2009;22:588–93.
2. Buvanendran A, Kroin JS, Berger RA, et al. Upregulation of prostaglandin E2 and interleukins in the central nervous system and peripheral tissue during and after surgery in humans. Anesthesiology 2006;104:403–10.
3. Graham GG, Scott KF. Mechanism of action of paracetamol. Am J Ther 2005;12: 46–55.
4. Göröcs TS, Lambert M, Rinne T, et al. Efficacy and tolerability of ready-to-use intravenous paracetamol solution as monotherapy or as adjunct analgesic therapy for postoperative pain in patients undergoing elective ambulatory surgery: open, prospective study. Int J Clin Pract 2009;63:112–20.
5. Salihoglu Z, Yildirim M, Demiroluk S, et al. Evaluation of intravenous paracetamol administration on postoperative pain and recovery characteristics in patients undergoing laparoscopic cholecystectomy. Surg Laparosc Endosc Percutan Tech 2009;19:321–3.
6. Wininger SJ, Miller H, Minkowitz HS, et al. A randomized, double-blind, placebo-controlled, repeated dose study of two intravenous acetaminophen dosing regimens for the treatment of pain after abdominal laparoscopic surgery. Clin Ther 2010;32:2348–69.
7. Sinatra RS, Jahr JS, Reynolds LW, et al. Efficacy and safety of single and repeated administration of 1 gram of intravenous acetaminophen injection (paracetamol) for pain management after major orthopedic surgery. Anesthesiology 2005;102:822–31.
8. Ender J, Borger MA, Scholz M, et al. Cardiac surgery fast-track treatment in a post-anesthetic care unit: six-month results of the Leipzig fast-track concept. Anesthesiology 2008;109(1):61–6.
9. Hong JY, Won Han S, Kim WO, et al. Fentanyl sparing effects of combined ketorolac and acetaminophen for outpatient inguinal hernia repair in children. J Urol 2010;183:1551–5.
10. Ong CK, Seymour RA, Lirk P, et al. Combining paracetamol (acetaminophen) with nonsteroidal antiinflammatory drugs: a qualitative systematic review of analgesic efficacy for acute postoperative pain. Anesth Analg 2010;110:1170–9.
11. Sun T, Sacan O, White PF, et al. Perioperative vs postoperative celecoxib on patient outcome after major plastic surgery procedures. Anesth Analg 2008; 106:950–8.
12. Southworth S, Peters J, Rock A, et al. A multicenter, randomized, double-blind, placebo-controlled trial of intravenous ibuprofen 400 and 800 mg every 6 hours in the management of postoperative pain. Clin Ther 2009;31(9):1922–35.
13. Grant GM, Mehlisch DR. Intranasal ketorolac for pain secondary to third molar impaction surgery: a randomized, double-blind, placebo-controlled trial. J Oral Maxillofac Surg 2010;68:1025–31.

14. Singla N, Fingla S, Minkowitz HS, et al. Intranasal ketorolac for acute postoperative pain. Curr Med Res Opin 2010;26(8):1915–23.
15. Massey T, Derry S, Moore RA, et al. Topical NSAIDs for acute pain in adults. Cochrane Database Syst Rev 2010;16(6):1–95.
16. National Institute for Health and Clinical Excellence. Osteoarthritis: the care and management of osteoarthritis in adults. NICE clinical guideline 59. Available at: http://www.nice.org.uk/nicemedia/pdf/CG59NICEguideline.pdf. Accessed March 21, 2011.
17. McCarberg BH, Argoff CE. Topical diclofenac epolamine patch 1.3% for treatment of acute pain caused by soft tissue injury. Int J Clin Pract 2010;64(11):1546–53.
18. Barthel HR, Haselwood D, Longley S III, et al. Randomized controlled trial of diclofenac sodium gel in knee osteoarthritis. Semin Arthritis Rheum 2009;39(3):203–12.
19. Moen MD. Topical diclofenac solution. Drugs 2009;69(18):2621–32.
20. Shainhouse JZ, Grierson LM, Naseer Z. A long-term, open-label study to confirm the safety of topical diclofenac solution containing dimethyl sulfoxide in the treatment of the osteoarthritic knee. Am J Ther 2010;17:566–76.
21. Galer BS. A comparative subjective assessment study of PENNSAID and Voltaren Gel, two topical formulations of diclofenac sodium. Pain Pract 2010;20:1–9.
22. Clarke H, Pereira S, Kennedy D, et al. Gabapentin decreases morphine consumption and improves functional recovery following total knee arthroplasty. Pain Res Manag 2009;14:217–22.
23. Rusy L, Hainsworth K, Nelson T, et al. Gabapentin use in pediatric spinal fusion patients: a randomized, double-blind, controlled trial. Anesth Analg 2010;110:1393–8.
24. Sen H, Sizlan A, Yanarates O, et al. A comparison of gabapentin and ketamine in acute and chronic pain after hysterectomy. Anesth Analg 2009;109:1645–50.
25. Khan ZH, Rahimi M, Makarem, et al. Optimal dose of pre-incision/post-incision gabapentin for pain relief following lumbar laminectomy: a randomized study. Acta Anaesthesiol Scand 2011;55:306–12.
26. Agarwal A, Gautam S, Gupta D, et al. Evaluation of a single preoperative dose of pregabalin for attenuation of postoperative pain after laparoscopic cholecystectomy. Br J Anaesth 2008;101:700–4.
27. Mathiesen O, Jacobsen LS, Holm HE, et al. Pregabalin and dexamethasone for postoperative pain control: a randomized controlled study in hip arthroplasty. Br J Anaesth 2008;101:535–41.
28. Buvanendran A, Kroin JS, Della Valle CJ, et al. Perioperative oral pregabalin reduces chronic pain after total knee arthroplasty: a prospective, randomized, controlled trial. Anesth Analg 2010;110:199–207.
29. Zhang J, Ho KY, Wang Y. Efficacy of pregabalin in acute postoperative pain: a meta-analysis. Br J Anaesth 2011;106:454–62.
30. Aasvang EK, Hansen JB, Malmstrom J, et al. The effect of wound instillation of a novel purified capsaicin formulation on postherniotomy pain: a double-blind, randomized, placebo-controlled study. Anesth Analg 2008;107:282–91.
31. Aasvang EK, Hansen JB, Kehlet H. Late sensory function after intraoperative capsaicin wound instillation. Acta Anaesthesiol Scand 2010;54:224–31.
32. Kissin I. Vanilloid-induced conduction analgesia: selective, dose-dependent, long lasting, with low level of potential neurotoxicity. Anesth Analg 2008;107:271–81.

33. Remerand F, Tendre CL, Baud A, et al. The early and delayed analgesic effects of ketamine after total hip arthroplasty: a prospective, randomized, controlled, double-blind study. Anesth Analg 2009;109(6):1963–71.

34. Loftus RW, Yeager MP, Clark JA, et al. Intraoperative ketamine reduces perioperative opiate consumption in opiate-dependent patients with chronic back pain undergoing back surgery. Anesthesiology 2010;113(3):639–46.

35. Schley M, Topfner S, Wiech K, et al. Continuous brachial plexus blockade in combination with the NMDA receptor antagonist memantine prevents phantom pain in acute traumatic upper limb amputees. Eur J Pain 2007;11:299–308.

36. Buvanendran A, McCarthy RJ, Kroin JS, et al. Intrathecal magnesium prolongs fentanyl analgesia: a prospective, randomized, controlled trial. Anesth Analg 2002;95:661–6.

37. Koinig H, Wallner T, Marhofer P, et al. Magnesium sulfate reduces intra- and postoperative analgesic requirements. Anesth Analg 1998;87:206–10.

38. Lena P, Balarac N, Lena D, et al. Fast track anesthesia with remifentanil and spinal analgesia for cardiac surgery: the effect on pain control and quality of recovery. J Cardiothorac Vasc Anesth 2008;22:536–42.

39. Tufanogullari B, White PF, Peixoto MP, et al. Dexmedetomidine infusion during laparoscopic bariatric surgery: the effect on recovery outcome variables. Anesth Analg 2008;106:1741–8.

40. Ramadhyani U, Park JL, Carollo DS, et al. Dexmedetomidine: clinical application as an adjunct for intravenous regional anesthesia. Anesthesiol Clin 2010;28:709–22.

41. Afilalo M, Stegmann JU, Upmalis D, et al. Tapentadol immediate release: a new treatment option for acute pain management. J Pain Res 2010;8:1–9.

42. Etropolski M, Kelly K, Okamoto A, et al. Comparable efficacy and superior gastrointestinal tolerability (nausea, vomiting, constipation) of tapentadol compared with oxycodone hydrochloride. Adv Ther 2011;28:401–17.

43. Kwong WJ, Ozer-Stillman I, Miller JD, et al. Cost-effectiveness analysis of tapentadol immediate release for the treatment of acute pain. Clin Ther 2010;32:1768–81.

44. Beaulieu P. Effects of nabilone, a synthetic cannabinoid, on postoperative pain. Can J Anaesth 2006;53:769–75.

# Pediatric Pain Management

Santhanam Suresh, MD*, Patrick K. Birmingham, MD,
Ryan J. Kozlowski, BS

**KEYWORDS**

- Pediatric anesthesia • Regional anesthesia • Nerve block
- Ultrasound and pediatric

Regional anesthesia has become an integral part of adult anesthesia. Although regional anesthesia is not routinely used in children because of the need for general anesthesia that is necessary to keep the patients from moving and cooperating with the operator, it has been gaining immense popularity in the last decade. Adjuvant pain medications, including opioids and nonsteroidal analgesics, have been used for managing pain postoperatively. In addition, there is always the fear of damaging nerves when regional anesthesia is performed in a child who is asleep and not able to physically respond to the needle placed intraneurally. Although there is not much objective evidence, both large prospective databases and expert opinion have demonstrated the ability to continue to perform regional anesthesia in the asleep child safely because major neural damage has not been reported in children.[1,2] A large database is currently maintained in North America (Pediatric Regional Anesthesia Network) that may shed light into the benefits, adverse effects, and feasibility of regional anesthesia in children (Santhanam Suresh, MD, personal communication, 2011). The use of ultrasonography and its introduction to the practice of regional anesthesia in children has markedly improved the application of regional anesthesia to routine pediatric anesthesia care. Methodical detailed systematic reviews of ultrasound-guided regional techniques are available for practitioners to apply to their routine practice.[3,4] The use of regional anesthesia and its application to every day practice has spawned because of data available to demonstrate decreased morbidity in children and better outcomes.[5] Teaching and providing hands-on dedicated pediatric regional anesthesia workshops at national meetings, including the American Society of Anesthesiology, the American Society for Regional Anesthesia and Pain

This work was supported by departmental funding.
Santhanam Suresh is supported by FAER Research in Education Grant and has equipment support from BK medical, Sonosite Inc. and Phillips Helathcare.
Department of Pediatric Anesthesiology, Children's Memorial Hospital, Northwestern University's Feinberg School of Medicine, 2300 Children's Plaza, Chicago, IL 60614, USA
* Corresponding author. Children's Memorial Hospital, 2300 Children's Plaza, Chicago, IL 60614.
*E-mail address:* ssuresh@childrensmemorial.org

Anesthesiology Clin 30 (2012) 101–117
doi:10.1016/j.anclin.2011.12.003
1932-2275/12/$ – see front matter © 2012 Published by Elsevier Inc.

Medicine (ASRA), and the Society for Pediatric Anesthesia (SPA), and the International Anesthesia Research Society (IARS) have provided platforms for gaining knowledge and dialogue amongst practitioners to increase their application of regional anesthesia in neonates, infants, children, and adolescents. This review discusses a comprehensive approach to acute pain management in infants, children, and adolescents.

## ASSESSMENT OF PAIN

Infants, toddlers, and younger children are unable or unwilling to verbalize or quantify pain like adults. Because of these cognitive or maturational differences, several developmentally appropriate pain assessment scales have been designed for use in either infants or children. These scales can be subdivided into validated self-report, behavioral, and/or physiologic measures. Children at approximately 8 to 10 years of age may be able to use the standard adult numeric rating or visual analog scale to self-report their pain. Specialized self-reporting scales such as the Bieri FACES scale[6] are available for children and can be used in patients as young as 3 to 4 years. Behavioral or physiologic measures are available for younger ages and for developmentally disabled children (**Table 1**). The FLACC (Face, Legs, Activity, Cry, Consolability) scale is one such behavioral scale that is widely used, easy to use, and validated.[7] The scale has also subsequently been revised (FLACC-R) for use in children with cognitive impairment.[8]

## THE ACUTE PAIN SERVICE

Hospital-based acute pain services have been established to coordinate and provide pain management in children and have become increasingly common over the past 2 decades. Although the structure of such services varies, in the United States these are largely organized and run by anesthesiology departments, often staffed by pediatric anesthesiologists, anesthesia fellows and residents, and/or pain nurse practitioners. With the success and proliferation of such services, they have expanded to cover painful nonsurgical conditions such as sickle cell disease and pediatric malignancies.

**Table 1**
**FLACC behavioral pain scale**

| Categories | Scoring 0 | Scoring 1 | Scoring 2 |
|---|---|---|---|
| Face | No expression or smile | Occasional grimace or frown, withdrawn and disinterested | Frequent constant frown, clenched jaw, quivering chin |
| Legs | Normal position or relaxed | Uneasy, restless, and tense | Kicking or legs drawn up |
| Activity | Lying quietly, normal position, moves easily | Squirming, shifting back and forth, tense | Arched, rigid, or jerking |
| Cry | No cry (awake or asleep) | Moans or whimpers, occasional complaint | Crying steadily, screams or sobs, frequent complaints |
| Consolability | Content, relaxed | Reassured by occasional touching, hugging, being talked to, distractible | Difficult to console or comfort |

*Data from* Merkel S, Voepel-Lewis T, Malviya S. Pain assessment in infants and young children: the FLACC scale. Am J Nurs 2002;102(10):55–8.

Most recently, there has been a focus on ensuring the continuity of pain management outside the hospital for the increasing number of children undergoing outpatient surgery.

## PATIENT-CONTROLLED ANALGESIA

Intravenous patient-controlled analgesia (PCA) is commonly and effectively used in children,[9] with more than 2 decades of accumulated published experience, research, and clinical studies to guide therapy. Alternative pro re nata (p.r.n.) or as-needed dosing potentially leads to cycles of pain interspersed with excessive sedation or other opioid-related side effects from the pro re nata rescue dosing. Indeed, PCA has been safely and effectively used in children as young as 5 to 6 years, with reports of "medically sophisticated" children as young as 2 years successfully using PCA. Compared with pro re nata intramuscular opioids, PCA has been shown to be safe in children and to provide more effective analgesia with greater patient satisfaction.[10] Morphine is the more frequently used and studied PCA opioid of choice. Hydromorphone and fentanyl are commonly used alternatives (**Table 2**). A continuous (aka background or basal) infusion is sometimes added for patients after major surgery to optimize analgesia. Opioid-related side effects are minimized with the use of lower-dose (eg, 0.01–0.02 mg/kg/h morphine) continuous infusions and are routinely used at our institution.[11]

The concept of PCA has been expanded to allow parent- or nurse-assisted analgesia in select cases in which the patient is unwilling or unable, because of age, developmental delay, or physical disability, to activate the PCA button. Although more commonly used in infants and children with cancer treatment–related pain, such as oral mucositis with bone marrow transplantation, it has been safely used for postoperative analgesia as well. Parent- or nurse-assisted initiation of PCA boluses has been safely used in patients younger than 1 year, with opioid-related side effects similar to those observed in older patients.[12] Respiratory depression occurred rarely but emphasizes the need for close monitoring and rescue protocols.

## EPIDURAL ANALGESIA

There are several differences in the performance of epidural analgesia in children versus adults. Often overlooked but deserving of brief mention is the issue of patient assent.[13] Assent is defined as a "child's affirmative agreement (preference) to participate" (National Committee for Protection of Human Subjects, 1977). Although there is no specific age mandate or cutoff at which a child's assent must be obtained, 10 to 12

| Table 2<br>PCA parameters[a] | | | |
|---|---|---|---|
| **Choice of Opioid** | **Morphine** | **Hydromorphone** | **Fentanyl** |
| Loading Dose (Over 1–5 min) | 0.05–0.20 mg/kg | 1–4 µg/kg | 0.5–2.0 µg/kg |
| Demand Dose | 0.01–0.02 mg/kg | 2–3 µg/kg | 0.2–0.4 µg/kg |
| Lockout Time (min) | 5–15 | 5–15 | 5–15 |
| 1-h Limit (Optional) | 0.10–0.20 mg/kg | 30–40 µg/kg | 3–4 µg/kg |
| Continuous Infusion (Optional) | 0.01–0.02 mg/kg/h | 2–3 µg/kg/h | 0.2–0.4 µg/kg/h |

[a] Dose ranges are approximate; selection of opioid and actual parameters depend on assessment of individual patient.

*Data from* Birmingham PK. Recent advances in acute pain management. Curr Probl Pediatr 1995;25:99–112.

years of age is used in most research protocols,[14] and the same practice can be applied toward the child undergoing epidural needle and/or catheter placement. In obtaining parental consent or patient assent, physician surveys indicate a tendency to routinely discuss common minor risks and rarely discuss severe major risks,[15] yet parent surveys indicate that 74% to 87% of parents want to know all the risks for their child, including the risk of death.[16] A recent prospective national pediatric epidural audit of more than 10,000 epidurals revealed an incidence of 1:2000 for serious complications, with an incidence of 1:10,000 for persisting sequelae at 12 months. No deaths or cardiac arrests were reported. More recently, a similar risk level was reported with opioids via PCA, nurse-controlled analgesia, and continuous opioid infusions.[17]

Another issue is whether an epidural is better administered in the awake versus anesthetized child. The practice of inserting epidural catheters in the awake adult patient is often not applicable to children, in whom sedation or general anesthesia is necessary to allow safe performance of regional anesthesia. It is accepted practice and has been the standard of care for many years to place epidurals in anesthetized children.[18] Recent practice advisory guidelines by the ASRA state, "The benefit of ensuring a cooperative and immobile infant or child may outweigh the risk of performing neuraxial regional anesthesia in pediatric patients undergoing general anesthesia or heavy sedation."[2]

Although chlorhexidine has been shown in children to reduce epidural catheter and insertion site colonization rates in comparison with povidone iodine, it is not approved for use in infants younger than 2 months because of concerns about skin irritation and/or absorption.[19]

In addition to differences in the termination of the spinal cord and dura mater in infants versus adults, the intercristal line surface landmark, connecting the posterior superior iliac spines, crosses the lumbar spine lower in infants, at the L5-S1 level versus the L3-L4 interspace in adults. Also, the depth of the epidural space from the lumbar skin varies more in children than in adults. Different formulas have been developed using body weight to calculate the distance (D) from the skin to the lumbar epidural space:

$$D \text{ (mm)} = (\text{weight in kg} + 10)\, 0.8$$

For example, in a 20-kg child the D would be calculated as follows: $(20 + 10)\, 0.8 = (30)\, 0.8 = 24$ mm = 2.4 cm distance to the epidural space. An alternative simpler approximation is D (mm) = 1 mm/kg body weight. So in the 20-kg child D would be 20 mm or 2 cm.[20] Because of the shorter distance relative to adults, a shorter epidural needle length is desirable and commercially available for use in children.

In infants and children up to approximately 5 years of age, it is possible to make use of the excellent caudal landmarks that are below the level of spinal cord termination to successfully thread catheters from the caudal epidural space to lumbar and lower thoracic levels[21,22] with the goal of placing the catheter tip close to the dermatomes desired for blockade. Catheter tip location can be verified by fluoroscopy with use of contrast media, electromyography, electrocardiography, or more recently ultrasonography.[23,24]

Before injection of a local anesthetic solution, the needle or catheter is inspected for passive blood or cerebrospinal fluid (CSF) return and then aspirated for blood or CSF. Because a negative aspirate may not guarantee correct needle or catheter position, an epidural test dose is given using local anesthetic and an intravascular marker such as epinephrine in a concentration of 1:200,000 (5 µg/mL) (**Box 1**).[25]

> **Box 1**
> **Epidural test dosing**
>
> - Local anesthetic, 0.1 mL/kg (maximum of 3 mL), with 1:200,000 epinephrine
> - Observation period of 60 seconds for any of the following 3 markers
>   - Heart rate increased by 10 beats per minute or more
>   - Systolic blood pressure increased by 10% or more
>   - T wave amplitude increased by 25% or more
> - Repeat procedure if equivocal

## CAUDAL BLOCKS

Caudal block is the most widely used pediatric regional technique for postoperative analgesia as a single-injection technique. Its popularity stems in part from the readily palpable landmarks and relative ease of caudal block insertion in infants and children compared with adults. Dosing formulae have been developed using age, weight, and number of spinal segments to be blocked. Weight is a better correlate in predicting spread and is more commonly used. Volumes of 0.5 to 1.0 mL/kg achieve blockade from L1 to T6 dermatomes, respectively.[26] Bupivacaine is the most commonly used local anesthetic, usually in a concentration of 0.125%. Duration of analgesia with bupivacaine, ropivacaine, and levobupivacaine is on average 4 to 6 hours. Clonidine is the most commonly used additive[27]; doses of 1 to 2 µg/kg of clonidine may enhance analgesia by 2 to 3 hours. Maximum initial dosing and approximate durations for commonly used local anesthetics is listed in **Table 3**.

## ADVERSE EFFECTS

Neurotoxicity such as seizures from a local anesthetic bolus or subsequent infusion can be treated with barbiturates, benzodiazepines, or propofol, although seizure activity can be masked under general anesthesia. Recent evidence indicates that the most successful treatment of local anesthetic cardiotoxicity is the use of lipid emulsion, which is now considered the first-line therapy.[28] Epinephrine in doses exceeding 10 µg/kg may actually impair lipid resuscitation (**Box 2**). A recent pediatric case report described successful resuscitation from ropivacaine/lidocaine-induced ventricular arrhythmias after posterior lumbar plexus block in a child.[29] There is a growing consensus that lipid emulsion be immediately available in cases in which regional anesthesia is administered.

**Table 3**
**Local anesthetic solution: suggested maximum initial dosing**

| Local Anesthetic Solution | Maximum Dose (mg/kg) | Duration of Action (h) |
|---|---|---|
| Bupivacaine | 2.5 | 3–6 |
| Ropivacaine | 3 | 2–4 |
| Levobupivacaine | 3 | 2–4 |
| Lidocaine | 7 | 1.5–2.5 |
| Chloroprocaine | 20 | 1.0–1.5 |

> **Box 2**
> **Treatment of local anesthetic toxicity**
>
> - Administer 1 mL/kg of 20% lipid emulsion over 1 minute
> - Repeat dose every 3 to 5 minutes to a maximum of 3 mL/kg
> - Maintenance infusion of 0.25 mL/kg/min under circulation restored
> - Propofol (10% lipid) is not a substitute

## Epidural Analgesia

Continuous epidural infusions via an indwelling catheter are used for extensive lower extremity orthopedic surgery, major abdominal procedures, and chest wall surgeries including thoracotomies.

Local anesthetic and additive solutions similar to those in adults are used in infants and children (**Table 4**). Lower infusion rates are generally recommended in neonates and infants younger than 3 to 6 months because of decreased plasma protein binding and consequently higher free (unbound) fractions of drug and pharmacokinetic differences, potentially resulting in higher plasma levels and prolonged drug half-life. Additives such as clonidine[30] may have a wider index of safety than previously thought. Three patients aged 14 months to 5 years received 100 times the intended dose of clonidine in single-dose caudal blocks. Although somnolence was reported, no respiratory depression, desaturation, or hemodynamic instability resulted.[31]

## Patient-Controlled Epidural Analgesia

The concept of PCA, well established with intravenous opioids, has been extended to epidural analgesia in children as well. Using parameters outlined in **Box 3**, patient-controlled epidural analgesia was used in 128 patients (132 procedures) as young as 5 years. Ninety percent of patients achieved satisfactory analgesia, with no patients requiring treatment of sedation or respiratory depression. More recently, the concept of parent/nurse-assisted epidural analgesia has been introduced to optimize dosing flexibility and pain relief given via the epidural route in patients unable to self-activate the demand dose button.[32] Results similar to the patient-controlled epidural

**Table 4**
**Suggested pediatric epidural dosing guidelines**

| Drug | Infusion Solution | Infusion Limits |
|------|-------------------|-----------------|
| Bupivacaine | 0.0625%–0.1% | ≤0.4–0.5 mg/kg/h |
| Ropivacaine | 0.1%–0.2% | ≤0.4–0.5 mg/kg/h |
| Fentanyl | 1–5 µg/mL | 0.5–2.0 µg/kg/h |
| Morphine | 5–10 µg/mL | 1–5 µg/kg/h |
| Hydromorphone | 2–5 µg/mL | 1.0–2.5 µg/kg/h |
| Clonidine | 0.5–1.0 µg/mL | 0.1–0.5 µg/kg/h |

These are approximate dose ranges. Actual dose selected depends on individual patient assessment. Infants younger than 3 to 6 months of age generally receive a 30% to 50% reduction in initial dosing and hourly infusion rates of local anesthetic or opioid.

*Data from* Malviya S, Polaner DM, Berde C. Acute pain. Chapter 44. In: Cote CJ, Lerman J, Todres ID, editors. A practice of anesthesia for infants and children. 4th edition. Philadelphia: Saunders Elsevier; 2009.

---

**Box 3**
**Patient-controlled epidural analgesia parameters**

- Administering 0.1% bupivacaine with 2 to 5 µg/mL fentanyl
- Starting infusion rate of 0.1 to 0.2 m/kg/h (thoracic catheter maximum, 8–10 mL/h) (lumbar catheter maximum, 12–15 mL/h)
- Demand dose of 0.5 to 2.0 mL
- A lockout of 15 to 30 minutes
- Hourly maximum (continuous + demand) of 0.4 mg/kg/h or less
- For example: in a 20-kg patient: 4 mL/h + 1 mL every 30 minutes = 6 mL/h (8 mL/h maximum allowed)

*Data from* Birmingham PK, Wheeler M, Suresh S, et al. Patient-controlled epidural analgesia in children: can they do it? Anesth Analg 2003;96(3):686–91.

---

analgesia group were obtained, with effective analgesia in 86% of patients and no patient requiring treatment of sedation or respiratory depression. The technique was used in patients as young as 5 months.

## PERIPHERAL NERVE BLOCKS

Peripheral nerve blockade has been growing in use as a means of providing regional anesthesia in the pediatric population. These nerve blocks are able to provide both intraoperative and postoperative analgesia and have also been shown to reduce postoperative nausea and vomiting in children.[1] The use of traditional regional anesthesia techniques has been challenging in infants and children because of the need to target neural structures that run very close to vessels and other critical structures,[3] but the addition of nerve stimulators and ultrasound guidance to the anesthesiologist's toolkit has expanded the potential for safe and effective use of peripheral nerve blockade in pediatric pain management. The indications for several commonly performed peripheral nerve blocks as well as a summary of the associated anatomy and techniques used for successful blockade are discussed (**Table 5**).

**Table 5**
**Peripheral nerve block: indications and dosing of bupivacaine 0.25%**

| Block | Indication | Dosing | Adverse Side Effects |
|---|---|---|---|
| Supraorbital | Craniotomy | 1–2 mL | Rare |
| Infraorbital | Cleft lips | 0.5–1 mL | Upper lip numbness, hematoma |
| Occipital | Craniotomy | 1–2 mL | Rare |
| Superficial cervical plexus | Mastoid surgery | 1–2 mL | Intravascular injection, hematoma |
| Brachial plexus | Upper extremity surgery | 0.3 mL/kg | Intravascular injection |
| Femoral nerve block | Femoral fractures | 0.3 mL/kg | Intravascular injection |
| Sciatic nerve | Foot surgery | 0.3 mL/kg | Intravascular injection |
| Transversus abdominis plane block | Abdominal surgery | 0.3 mL/kg per side | Rare |
| Ilioinguinal nerve | Hernia surgery | 0.1 mL/kg | Rare |
| Rectus sheath | Umbilical hernia | 0.1 mL/kg | Rare, hematoma |

## HEAD AND NECK NERVE BLOCKS

Head and neck nerve blocks are particularly useful for postoperative pain control in pediatric patients. Often, these blocks can be successfully completed using the landmark techniques outlined later.

### Supraorbital Nerve

The supraorbital nerve is the first division of the trigeminal nerve as it exits the supraorbital foramen and supplies the forehead and the area anterior to the coronal suture. This block is indicated for surgery on the forehead, including craniotomy. We have used this block successfully for infants undergoing Ommaya placement without the use of general anesthesia.[33]

### Technique

After sterile preparation, a 30-gauge needle is inserted at the level of the supraorbital foramen, which is usually located in the midpupillary line in the eyebrow. The local anesthetic solution is injected subcutaneously to provide analgesia for the forehead (**Fig. 1**).

### Infraorbital Nerve

The second division of the trigeminal nerve exits the infraorbital foramen and supplies the maxillary area. This nerve is usually blocked to provide analgesia for sinus surgery[34] and cleft lip repairs.[35]

### Technique

An intraoral approach to the infraorbital nerve is preferred in our institution. After eversion of the lip, a 27-gauge needle is inserted with the needle trajectory toward the infraorbital foramen; after aspiration, 0.5 mL to 2.0 mL is injected to provide analgesia for the upper lip and the maxilla (**Fig. 2**).

### Occipital Nerve

The greater occipital nerve is derived off the C2 nerve root to supply the occipital portion of the scalp. This supply is used for managing patients with occipital neuralgia as well as in patients with transformed migraines.[36] This can also be used in patients with postoperative pain after posterior fossa craniotomies. The occipital nerve can be

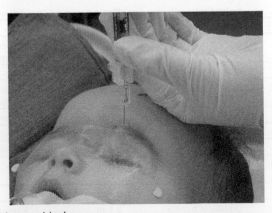

**Fig. 1.** Supraorbital nerve block.

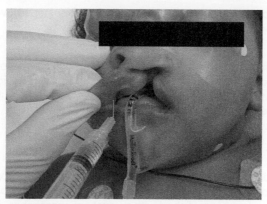

**Fig. 2.** Infraorbital nerve block.

identified in the posterior fossa below the nuchal line situated near the occipital artery. More recent findings for occipital nerve blocks with the use of ultrasonography can facilitate accurate placement of these blocks.[37]

### Technique

After palpation of the occipital protuberance, the finger is slid down and the occipital artery palpated; the nerve is located medial to the artery caudad of the superior nuchal line and lateral to the artery superiorly. Alternatively, using ultrasound guidance, the C2 transverse process is located. The probe is then tilted cephalad and the obliquus capitis muscle identified. The greater occipital nerve is noted to be on top of the obliquus capitis muscle in this position. Local anesthetic is injected into the area of the nerve (**Fig. 3**).

### Superficial Cervical Plexus

The superficial cervical plexus is derived off the cervical roots C3 and C4. The superficial cervical plexus wraps around the belly of the sternocleidomastoid and sends out 3 branches: the lesser occipital nerve, the great auricular nerve, and the transverse cervical and supraclavicular nerve. A blockade of the great auricular nerve can provide

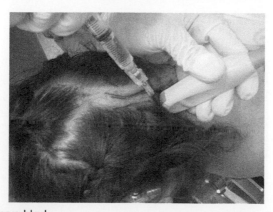

**Fig. 3.** Occipital nerve block.

analgesia for the postauricular area and can facilitate postoperative pain control in children undergoing tympanomastoid surgery.[5]

### Technique

After sterile preparation, the lateral border of the sternocleidomastoid is identified at the level of the cricoid cartilage (C6). A needle is placed, with the injection administered subcutaneously; injecting 2 mL of the local anesthetic solution can provide adequate analgesia for postoperative pain control (**Fig. 4**).

## UPPER EXTREMITY BLOCKS

Peripheral nerve blockade can be useful in providing analgesia for both open and closed surgical procedures of the upper extremity in the pediatric population. Upper extremity blocks can be accomplished with a variety of approaches, including axillary, interscalene, supraclavicular, and infraclavicular. These blocks may be safer and more effective when using ultrasonography to visualize the pertinent anatomy during administration of the nerve block.[3]

### Axillary Approach

The axillary approach is the most commonly performed brachial plexus block in children.[38] This technique is indicated for surgical procedures on the elbow, forearm, or hand because the axillary approach blocks the radial, median, and ulnar nerves. With the arm abducted and externally rotated, the probe is placed perpendicular to the axillary fold, and the branches of the brachial plexus can be seen surrounding the axillary artery, superficially between the biceps muscle and humerus. The musculocutaneous nerve can exit the axillary sheath proximal to the placement of this block; so if the biceps or forearm is involved in the surgical procedure, blocking the musculocutaneous nerve within the belly of the coracobrachialis is recommended in addition to blocking the axillary brachial plexus.[3]

### Technique

The arm is abducted, a linear ultrasound probe is placed in the axilla, the nerves surrounding the axillary artery are identified, and the local anesthetic solution is injected to block each one of the individual branches, including the median, radial,

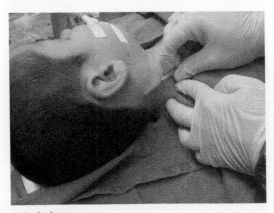

**Fig. 4.** Superficial cervical plexus.

ulnar, and musculocutaneous nerves. Care has to be taken to ensure that the needle is not placed in the artery.

### Interscalene Approach

The interscalene approach is indicated for surgical procedures on the shoulder, upper arm, and elbow because the interscalene approach blocks the C5, C6, and C7 nerve roots between the anterior and middle scalene muscles.

#### Technique

A small footprint, high-frequency probe is placed at the posterolateral aspect of the sternocleidomastoid muscle in a transverse oblique plane at the level of the cricoid cartilage. The brachial plexus can be visualized as a hyperechoic structure in the interscalene groove posterior to the sternocleidomastoid muscle, and a needle can be advanced and local anesthetic delivered into the space surrounding the plexus for blockade.

### Supraclavicular Approach

The supraclavicular approach is indicated for most surgical procedures of the upper extremity, including procedures of the upper arm and elbow, because this approach blocks the trunks and divisions of the brachial plexus as it courses just anterior and lateral to the first rib.

#### Technique

The probe is placed lateral and superior to the clavicle, in a coronal oblique plane, and the brachial plexus is visualized superior and lateral to the subclavian artery.[39] A needle is inserted lateral to the probe, advanced in plane, and directed medially to deliver local anesthetic. This can be performed using ultrasound guidance for postoperative pain control after checking the integrity of the nerves after upper extremity fracture reductions.[40]

### Infraclavicular Approach

The infraclavicular approach is indicated for surgical procedures of the arm, elbow, and forearm because this approach blocks the cords of the brachial plexus as they course lateral, posterior, and medial to the axillary artery.[41]

#### Technique

A high-frequency probe is placed in a parasagittal plane immediately medial and inferior to the coracoid process, and the brachial plexus is seen as 3 cords surrounding the axillary artery. A needle is inserted inferomedially to the coracoid process with an in-plane approach, advanced through pectoralis major and minor, and aimed at the hyperechoic posterior cord of the brachial plexus.[39] After aspiration, the local anesthetic solution is injected and the spread of the local anesthetic is visualized. This block may be performed without the aid of neurostimulation in patients with fractures.

## LOWER EXTREMITY BLOCKS

Regional anesthesia of the lower extremity can be achieved by peripheral nerve blockade of the lumbar plexus, femoral, or sciatic nerves. The lumbar plexus consists of lumbar nerves L1 through L4 and gives rise to the femoral nerve, the lateral femoral cutaneous nerve, and the obturator nerve, whereas the sciatic nerve is derived from the sacral plexus, which consists of the anterior rami of L4 through S3.

### Lumbar Plexus

Blockade of the lumbar plexus is indicated for surgical procedures of the hip, pelvis, leg, or foot because this approach blocks the femoral, genitofemoral, lateral femoral cutaneous, and obturator nerves. A low-frequency probe is used to visualize the lumbar plexus because of its depth. The probe is placed on a longitudinal axis lateral to the spinous processes to visualize the transverse processes of L4 or L5. The probe is then rotated to the transverse axis, and the lumbar plexus is visualized within the psoas major muscle below the erector spinae and quadratus lumborum muscles.[42] The needle is advanced in plane, and the injected local anesthetic should be seen spreading within the posterior part of the psoas major.

### Femoral Nerve

Femoral nerve blocks are indicated for surgical procedures on the anterior thigh and knee because this approach targets the nerve as it courses lateral to the femoral artery and blocks the areas of the lower extremity supplied by nerve roots L2, L3, and L4.

#### Technique

The ultrasound probe is placed parallel and inferior to the inguinal ligament, and the nerve is visualized lateral to the femoral artery.[43] The needle can then be advanced in or out of plane, and local anesthetic is injected while adequate spread is visualized.

### Sciatic Nerve

The sciatic nerve block is indicated for surgical procedures of the leg, foot, and ankle, and anesthetic can be administered by either a subgluteal approach or a popliteal fossa approach. The subgluteal approach blocks the sciatic nerve proximal to its bifurcation into the common peroneal and tibial nerves.

#### Technique

A low-frequency curvilinear probe is used to ensure visualization at the depth of the sciatic nerve between the ischial tuberosity and the greater trochanter. A probe is placed transversely below the gluteal fold, and the sciatic nerve can be visualized in cross section deep to the gluteus maximus muscle.[43] The needle is inserted in plane, and the spread of local anesthetic solution is visualized.

The popliteal fossa approach blocks the sciatic nerve as it bifurcates to form the common peroneal and tibial nerves. A probe can be positioned transversely at the popliteal crease, and the anesthesiologist can visualize the common peroneal nerve lateral and the tibial nerve posterior to the popliteal vein and artery. The probe is then moved cephalad to visualize the point of bifurcation, and the sciatic nerve appears as a large round hyperechoic structure proximal to this point. The needle may be placed in or out of plane and local anesthetic injected under ultrasound guidance.

### Truncal

Regional anesthestic techniques for peripheral nerve blockade of the anterior trunk are increasingly used to provide anesthesia during surgical procedures of the inguinal, umbilical, and epigastric regions.

#### Transversus abdominis plane

The transversus abdominis plane block is indicated for surgical procedures on the abdomen because the transversus abdominis plane is a potential space between the internal oblique and transversus abdominis muscle, which contains the thoracolumbar nerve roots T8 through L1.

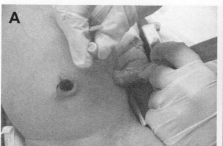
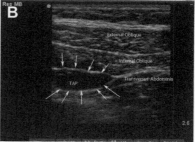

Fig. 5. (*A, B*) Transversus abdominis plane (TAP) block. The arrows point out to the nerves.

**Technique** A high-frequency probe is placed on the abdomen lateral to the umbilicus, and the 3 layers of the abdominal wall are identified. A needle is inserted through the external and internal oblique muscles, into the plane between the internal oblique and transversus abdominis muscle.[44] Local anesthetic injection creates an elliptical opening of the potential space (**Fig. 5**).

### Ilioinguinal
The ilioinguinal nerve block is indicated for surgical procedures in the lower abdomen and inguinal region, such as hernia repair and groin surgery, because the ilioinguinal and iliohypogastric nerves are the terminal branches of the L1 nerve root, which run through the transversus abdominis plane and supply the inguinal region.[45]

**Technique** A high-frequency probe is placed medial to the anterior superior iliac spine with the axis facing the umbilicus. A needle is inserted toward the ilioinguinal nerve as it runs between the transversus abdominis and internal oblique, and the anesthetic solution is injected under visualization (**Fig. 6**). More recently, the use of ilioinguinal nerve block in addition to the use of caudal blocks was examined in children undergoing groin surgery; it was demonstrated to be more useful in children undergoing inguinal hernia surgery than other groin procedures.[46]

### Rectus sheath
The rectus sheath block is indicated for surgical procedures of the umbilicus and superficial abdomen because the space between the rectus abdominis muscle and

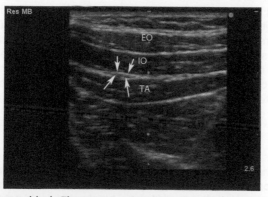

Fig. 6. Ilioinguinal nerve block. The arrows point out to the nerves. EO, external oblique; IO, internal oblique; TA, transversus abdominis.

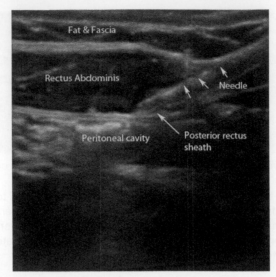

**Fig. 7.** Rectus sheath block. The arrows point out to the nerves.

the posterior rectus sheath contains the anterior abdominal branches of the intercostals nerves.

**Technique** A high-frequency probe is placed below the umbilicus and above the arcuate line.[47] The anterior and posterior walls of the rectus sheath are visualized superficial and deep to the rectus abdominis muscle. A needle is inserted through the muscle, and the anesthetic solution is injected into the potential space between the rectus abdominis and the posterior wall of the rectus sheath (**Fig. 7**). This is more useful for children undergoing single-incision laparoscopic procedures or for umbilical hernia repairs.[48]

## CONTINUOUS NERVE BLOCK CATHETERS

Continuous nerve block catheters are used in children more frequently than ever before. The use of nerve catheters has decreased the need for hospitalization after major surgery and has decreased the incidence of morbidity, including postoperative nausea and vomiting.[49] Most common catheters used include upper and lower extremity catheters for either the brachial plexus or the femoral and sciatic nerves. Clear instructions should be provided for discharge, including the need for assistance during ambulation if a lower extremity catheter is used. Recently we have started using ilioinguinal nerve catheters for iliac bone grafts[50] as well as transverse abdominis plane block catheters for children who have spinal dysraphism who may not be candidates for epidural or spinal anesthesia.[51]

## SUMMARY

Pediatric pain management has undergone some bold changes in the last 2 decades. The introduction of ultrasound guidance has clearly improved the ability to perform common blocks, particularly the use of truncal blocks that could not otherwise be performed in this group of patients without fear of visceral damage. Important work in this area, including pharmacokinetic work, has to be performed to demonstrate adequate safety of these parameters in infants and children. Introduction of newer drugs, particularly analgesics, has been usually overlooked in children; however, a new Food and Drug Administration mandate allows for the study and use of these drugs that are commonly used in adults to be used in children, allowing the armamentarium to expand rapidly. The old adage that pain in children is a myth is now replaced with the new slogan that pain in children has to be addressed adequately as in the practice in adults. More clinical trials using a variety of algorithms for managing pain in infants and children and adolescents will become available in the next decade.

## REFERENCES

1. Giaufre E, Dalens B, Gombert A. Epidemiology and morbidity of regional anesthesia in children: a one-year prospective survey of the French-Language Society of Pediatric Anesthesiologists. Anesth Analg 1996;83(5):904–12.
2. Bernards CM, Hadzic A, Suresh S, et al. Regional anesthesia in anesthetized or heavily sedated patients. Reg Anesth Pain Med 2008;33(5):449–60.
3. Tsui B, Suresh S. Ultrasound imaging for regional anesthesia in infants, children, and adolescents: a review of current literature and its application in the practice of extremity and trunk blocks. Anesthesiology 2010;112(2):473–92.
4. Tsui BC, Suresh S. Ultrasound imaging for regional anesthesia in infants, children, and adolescents: a review of current literature and its application in the practice of neuraxial blocks. Anesthesiology 2010;112(3):719–28.
5. Suresh S, Barcelona SL, Young NM, et al. Postoperative pain management in children undergoing tympanomastoid surgery: is a local block better than intravenous opioids? Anesthesiology 1999;91(3A):A1281.
6. Bieri D, Reeve RA, Champion GD, et al. The Faces Pain Scale for the self-assessment of the severity of pain experienced by children: development, initial validation and preliminary investigation for ratio scale properties. Pain 1990;41: 139–50.
7. Merkel S, Voepel-Lewis T, Malviya S. Pain assessment in infants and young children: the FLACC scale. Am J Nurs 2002;102(10):55–8.
8. Malviya S, Voepel-Lewis T, Tait AR, et al. Pain management in children with and without cognitive impairment following spine fusion surgery. Paediatr Anaesth 2001;11(4):453–8.
9. Berde CB, Sethna NF. Analgesics for the treatment of pain in children. N Engl J Med 2002;347(14):1094–103.
10. Berde CB, Beyer JE, Bournaki MC, et al. Comparison of morphine and methadone for prevention of postoperative pain in 3- to 7-year-old children. J Pediatr 1991;119(1 Pt 1):136–41.
11. Nelson KL, Yaster M, Kost-Byerly S, et al. A national survey of American Pediatric Anesthesiologists: patient-controlled analgesia and other intravenous opioid therapies in pediatric acute pain management. Anesth Analg 2010;110(3):754–60.
12. Monitto CL, Greenberg RS, Kost-Byerly S, et al. The safety and efficacy of parent-/nurse-controlled analgesia in patients less than six years of age. Anesth Analg 2000;91(3):573–9.
13. Lonnqvist PA, Morton NS, Ross AK. Consent issues and pediatric regional anesthesia. Paediatr Anaesth 2009;19(10):958–60.
14. Tait AR, Voepel-Lewis T, Malviya S. Do they understand? (part II): assent of children participating in clinical anesthesia and surgery research. Anesthesiology 2003;98(3):609–14.

15. Brull R, McCartney CJ, Chan VW, et al. Disclosure of risks associated with regional anesthesia: a survey of academic regional anesthesiologists. Reg Anesth Pain Med 2007;32(1):7–11.
16. Litman RS, Perkins FM, Dawson SC. Parental knowledge and attitudes toward discussing the risk of death from anesthesia. Anesth Analg 1993;77(2):256–60.
17. Morton NS, Errera A. APA national audit of pediatric opioid infusions. Paediatr Anaesth 2010;20(2):119–25.
18. Krane EJ, Dalens BJ, Murat I, et al. The safety of epidurals placed during general anesthesia. Reg Anesth Pain Med 1998;23(5):433–8.
19. Kinirons B, Mimoz O, Lafendi L, et al. Chlorhexidine versus povidone iodine in preventing colonization of continuous epidural catheters in children: a randomized, controlled trial. Anesthesiology 2001;94(2):239–44.
20. Suresh S, Wheeler M. Practical pediatric regional anesthesia. Anesthesiol Clin North Am 2002;20(1):83–113.
21. Bosenberg AT, Bland BA, Schulte-Steinberg O, et al. Thoracic epidural anesthesia via caudal route in infants. Anesthesiology 1988;69(2):265–9.
22. Tsui BC, Seal R, Entwistle L. Thoracic epidural analgesia via the caudal approach using nerve stimulation in an infant with CATCH22. Can J Anaesth 1999;46(12): 1138–42.
23. Tsui BC, Guenther C, Emery D, et al. Determining epidural catheter location using nerve stimulation with radiological confirmation. Reg Anesth Pain Med 2000; 25(3):306–9.
24. Willschke H, Bosenberg A, Marhofer P, et al. Epidural catheter placement in neonates: sonoanatomy and feasibility of ultrasonographic guidance in term and preterm neonates. Reg Anesth Pain Med 2007;32(1):34–40.
25. Polaner D, Suresh S, Cote CJ, et al. Pediatric regional anesthesia. In: Cote CJ, Todres ID, Goudsouzian NG, et al, editors. A practice of anesthesia for infants and children, vol. 3. Philadelphia: WB Saunders Company; 2000. p. 636–75.
26. Takasaki M, Dohi S, Kawabata Y, et al. Dosage of lidocaine for caudal anesthesia in infants and children. Anesthesiology 1977;47(6):527–9.
27. Menzies R, Congreve K, Herodes V, et al. A survey of pediatric caudal extradural anesthesia practice. Paediatr Anaesth 2009;19(9):829–36.
28. Weinberg G. Lipid rescue resuscitation from local anaesthetic cardiac toxicity. Toxicol Rev 2006;25(3):139–45.
29. Ludot H, Tharin JY, Belouadah M, et al. Successful resuscitation after ropivacaine and lidocaine-induced ventricular arrhythmia following posterior lumbar plexus block in a child. Anesth Analg 2008;106(5):1572–4.
30. Birmingham PK, Wheeler M, Suresh S, et al. Patient-controlled epidural analgesia in children: can they do it? Anesth Analg 2003;96(3):686–91, Table of Contents.
31. Meyer C, Cambray R. One hundred times the intended dose of caudal clonidine in three pediatric patients. Paediatr Anaesth 2008;18(9):888–90.
32. Birmingham PK, Suresh S, Ambrosy A, et al. Parent-assisted or nurse-assisted epidural analgesia: is this feasible in pediatric patients? Paediatr Anaesth 2009;19(11):1084–9.
33. Uejima T, Suresh S. Ommaya and McComb reservoir placement in infants: can this be done with regional anesthesia? Paediatr Anaesth 2008;18(9): 909–11.
34. Higashizawa T, Koga Y. Effect of infraorbital nerve block under general anesthesia on consumption of isoflurane and postoperative pain in endoscopic endonasal maxillary sinus surgery. J Anesth 2001;15(3):136–8.

35. Simion C, Corcoran J, Iyer A, et al. Postoperative pain control for primary cleft lip repair in infants: is there an advantage in performing peripheral nerve blocks? Paediatr Anaesth 2008;18(11):1060–5.

36. Ashkenazi A, Matro R, Shaw JW, et al. Greater occipital nerve block using local anaesthetics alone or with triamcinolone for transformed migraine: a randomised comparative study. J Neurol Neurosurg Psychiatry 2008;79(4):415–7.

37. Eichenberger U, Greher M, Kapral S, et al. Sonographic visualization and ultrasound-guided block of the third occipital nerve: prospective for a new method to diagnose C2-C3 zygapophysial joint pain. Anesthesiology 2006; 104(2):303–8.

38. Fleischmann E, Marhofer P, Greher M, et al. Brachial plexus anaesthesia in children: lateral infraclavicular vs axillary approach. Paediatr Anaesth 2003;13(2): 103–8.

39. De Jose Maria B, Banus E, Navarro Egea M, et al. Ultrasound-guided supraclavicular vs infraclavicular brachial plexus blocks in children. Paediatr Anaesth 2008;18(9):838–44.

40. Suresh S, Sarwark JP, Bhalla T, et al. Performing US-guided nerve blocks in the postanesthesia care unit (PACU) for upper extremity fractures: is this feasible in children? Paediatr Anaesth 2009;19(12):1238–40.

41. Marhofer P, Sitzwohl C, Greher M, et al. Ultrasound guidance for infraclavicular brachial plexus anaesthesia in children. Anaesthesia 2004;59(7):642–6.

42. Kirchmair L, Enna B, Mitterschiffthaler G, et al. Lumbar plexus in children. A sonographic study and its relevance to pediatric regional anesthesia. Anesthesiology 2004;101(2):445–50.

43. Oberndorfer U, Marhofer P, Bosenberg A, et al. Ultrasonographic guidance for sciatic and femoral nerve blocks in children. Br J Anaesth 2007;98(6):797–801.

44. Suresh S, Chan VW. Ultrasound guided transversus abdominis plane block in infants, children and adolescents: a simple procedural guidance for their performance. Paediatr Anaesth 2009;19(4):296–9.

45. Willschke H, Marhofer P, Bosenberg A, et al. Ultrasonography for ilioinguinal/iliohypogastric nerve blocks in children. Br J Anaesth 2005;95(2):226–30.

46. Jagannathan N, Sohn L, Sawardekar A, et al. Unilateral groin surgery in children: will the addition of an ultrasound-guided ilioinguinal nerve block enhance the duration of analgesia of a single-shot caudal block? Paediatr Anaesth 2009; 19(9):892–8.

47. de Jose Maria B, Gotzens V, Mabrok M. Ultrasound-guided umbilical nerve block in children: a brief description of a new approach. Paediatr Anaesth 2007;17(1): 44–50.

48. Rozen WM, Tran TM, Ashton MW, et al. Refining the course of the thoracolumbar nerves: a new understanding of the innervation of the anterior abdominal wall. Clin Anat 2008;21(4):325–33.

49. Ganesh A, Rose JB, Wells L, et al. Continuous peripheral nerve blockade for inpatient and outpatient postoperative analgesia in children. Anesth Analg 2007;105(5):1234–42.

50. Isyanov A, Suresh S. Continuous ilioinguinal nerve catheter infusions for iliac bone graft: postoperative pain control without adverse effects! Paediatr Anaesth 2009;19(3):282–3.

51. Taylor LJ, Birmingham P, Yerkes E, et al. Children with spinal dysraphism: transversus abdominis plane (TAP) catheters to the rescue! Paediatr Anaesth 2010; 20(10):951–4.

# Index

*Note:* Page numbers of article titles are in **boldface** type.

### A

Acetaminophen, injectable, in multimodal analgesia, 91–92
Acute pain service, hospital-based, for pediatric patients, 102–103
Alpha-2 agonists, in multimodal analgesia, 96
American Board of Surgery, role in recognition of palliative surgical care, 24
American College of Surgeons, role in recognition of palliative surgical care, 22–24
Analgesia. *See* Pain management.
Anatomy, for paravertebral blocks, 75–76
Anesthesia, regional, for pediatric pain management, **101–117**
    adverse effects, 105–107
    assessment of pain, 102
    caudal blocks, 105
    continuous nerve block catheters, 114
    epidural analgesia, 103–105
    head and neck nerve blocks, 108–110
    hospital-based acute pain services, 102–103
    lower extremity blocks, 111–114
    patient controlled analgesia, 103
    peripheral nerve blocks, 107
    upper extremity blocks, 110–111
Anesthetics, long-acting local, in multimodal analgesia, 97
Anticonvulsants, in multimodal analgesia, 94
Assessment, of pain in pediatric patients, 102

### B

Bereavement, support of the family in the surgical intensive care unit, 38–39

### C

Cannabinoids, in multimodal analgesia, 97
Capsaicin, in multimodal analgesia, 94–95
Cardiopulmonary resuscitation (CPR), in palliative surgery in the DNR patient, **1–12**
Caudal blocks, in pediatric patients, 107
Communication, as core skill of palliative surgical care, **47–58**
    improving skills in, 53–56
    in the perioperative period, 51–53
  in care of families in the surgical intensive care unit, **37–46**
    family as surrogate decision maker, 39–41
    grief and bereavement, 38–39
    interventions for, 43–44

Anesthesiology Clin 30 (2012) 119–125
doi:10.1016/S1932-2275(12)00015-8
1932-2275/12/$ – see front matter © 2012 Elsevier Inc. All rights reserved.
anesthesiology.theclinics.com

# Moving?

## Make sure your subscription moves with you!

To notify us of your new address, find your **Clinics Account Number** (located on your mailing label above your name), and contact customer service at:

Email: journalscustomerservice-usa@elsevier.com

800-654-2452 (subscribers in the U.S. & Canada)
314-447-8871 (subscribers outside of the U.S. & Canada)

Fax number: 314-447-8029

Elsevier Health Sciences Division
Subscription Customer Service
3251 Riverport Lane
Maryland Heights, MO 63043

*To ensure uninterrupted delivery of your subscription, please notify us at least 4 weeks in advance of move.

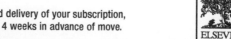

# Moving?

## Make sure your subscription moves with you!

To notify us of your new address, find your Clinics Account Number (located on your mailing label above your name), and contact customer service at:

Email: journalscustomerservice-usa@elsevier.com

800-654-2452 (subscribers in the U.S. & Canada)
314-447-8871 (subscribers outside of the U.S. & Canada)

Fax number: 314-447-8029

Elsevier Health Sciences Division
Subscription Customer Service
3251 Riverport Lane
Maryland Heights, MO 63043

Printed and bound by CPI Group (UK) Ltd, Croydon, CR0 4YY

03/10/2024

01040454-0010